Governing Human-Centric AI in Healthcare

The debate about artificial intelligence (AI) in healthcare is no longer focused on whether AI will be used, but on how it should be governed. Across Europe and beyond, policymakers, healthcare organizations, and technology developers are searching for ways to ensure that AI systems remain accountable, transparent, and aligned with human values. The European Union's Artificial Intelligence Act represents one of the most ambitious attempts to address these challenges through a human-centric approach. Yet an important question remains unanswered: what does human-centric AI actually look like when organizations begin implementing AI technologies in practice?

This book explores that question in the context of healthcare and humanoid robotics. Rather than examining regulation or technology in isolation, it brings together perspectives from AI governance, management, healthcare, and technology acceptance research. The discussion moves from the principles embedded in the AI Act to the realities of organizational decision-making, showing how ideas such as human dignity, human oversight, trust, inclusivity, and accountability influence the adoption of emerging technologies.

A central theme running throughout the book is the gap between technological possibility and organizational readiness. Drawing on empirical research involving 527 respondents – current and future decision-makers, the book examines perceptions of humanoid robots in healthcare and identifies the factors that encourage or discourage their adoption. The findings reveal that acceptance is shaped not only by expected benefits but also by concerns about trust, responsibility, ethics, patient safety, and the preservation of human interaction in care.

The book also proposes two original concepts: the Human-Centric Robot Acceptance Index (HCRAI), which evaluates readiness for humanoid robot adoption, and the Risk Gradient Model of Humanoid Robot Task Acceptance, which explains why some healthcare tasks are considered more suitable for robots than others. Together, these contributions offer new ways of understanding how AI technologies can be integrated into healthcare organizations while maintaining meaningful human oversight.

Written for researchers, healthcare professionals, managers, policymakers, and students, this book provides an interdisciplinary perspective on one of the most important challenges facing contemporary healthcare: ensuring that technological innovation remains centered on people rather than technology itself.

Ida Skubis is an Assistant Professor at Silesian University of Technology, Poland. She holds a PhD and four master's degrees. Dr. Ida Skubis is an AI researcher and linguist who combines extensive academic and managerial experience. She has received prestigious fellowships in France and Israel, and the Polish Minister's Scholarship for Outstanding Young Scientists. Her research focuses on AI ethics, digital health, and human-centric AI.

Governing Human-Centric AI in Healthcare

Acceptance, Risk, and Managerial Decision Models for Humanoid Robots

Ida Skubis

CRC Press
Taylor & Francis Group
Boca Raton London New York

CRC Press is an imprint of the
Taylor & Francis Group, an informa business

First edition published 2027
by CRC Press
2385 NW Executive Center Drive, Suite 320, Boca Raton FL 33431

and by CRC Press
4 Park Square, Milton Park, Abingdon, Oxon, OX14 4RN

CRC Press is an imprint of Taylor & Francis Group, LLC

ISBN: 9781041413646 (hbk)
ISBN: 9781041413707 (pbk)
ISBN: 9781042027200 (ebk)

DOI: 10.1201/9781042027200

Typeset in Times
by Newgen Publishing UK

Contents

Introduction

Artificial intelligence shapes high-stakes domains, including healthcare, where automated or semi-automated systems promise efficiency gains, improved logistics, and new forms of clinical support. At the same time, these systems introduce ethical and societal risks: bias, opacity, privacy vulnerabilities, and the erosion of human agency, especially when decisions affect fundamental rights, personal autonomy, and human dignity. The central governance challenge is therefore not merely how to accelerate innovation but how to ensure that innovation remains human-centric: aligned with societal values, protective of rights, and responsive to the lived realities of people who experience technology directly.

Healthcare provides a particularly important context for examining these challenges. AI systems are increasingly used in diagnostics, patient monitoring, administrative processes, rehabilitation, and decision-support systems, while social and humanoid robots are gradually entering hospitals, care facilities, and service environments. Although these technologies offer opportunities to improve efficiency and service quality, they also raise questions concerning trust, transparency, accountability, privacy, and human oversight (Floridi et al., 2018; Dignum, 2019; Shneiderman, 2020). As AI systems become more deeply embedded in professional environments, the challenge increasingly concerns not only technological capabilities but also effective forms of human–AI collaboration and responsible integration into organizational processes (Skubis et al. 2026).

The European Commission and EU institutions have developed one of the most influential global approaches to AI governance, combining ethical guidance with binding legal obligations. The Artificial Intelligence Act (AI Act) represents a landmark effort to translate ethical principles, such as trust, accountability, transparency, fairness, and human oversight, into a risk-based regulatory framework. Yet the existence of a regulatory framework does not guarantee that its human-centric ideals will be realized in practice. Implementation depends on the choices of organizations and the people who manage them: what technologies are adopted, how responsibilities are assigned, which safeguards are designed, and how human oversight is ensured throughout the system lifecycle.

DOI: 10.1201/9781042027200-1

This book addresses a critical gap: the connection between human-centric AI as a legal-ethical project and human-centric AI as an organizational-managerial practice. Many studies examine policy and regulation, while others analyze adoption and acceptance of AI systems within organizations. Fewer works explicitly connect these levels and show how the language of human-centric governance is interpreted, operationalized, or resisted in real-world decision-making, especially in sensitive sectors such as healthcare, where trust and human contact are integral to care itself.

The discussion is grounded in several complementary theoretical perspectives. Human-Centered Artificial Intelligence emphasizes the need to combine technological capabilities with meaningful human control and oversight (Shneiderman, 2020). Technology Acceptance Model research demonstrates that perceived usefulness and perceived ease of use play central roles in shaping technology adoption (Davis, 1989), while the Diffusion of Innovations theory highlights the importance of knowledge, persuasion, and organizational legitimacy during implementation processes (Rogers, 2003). The Socio-Technical Systems theory further suggests that successful implementation depends not only on technical performance but also on the alignment of technologies with organizational structures, professional practices, and social expectations (Trist & Bamforth, 1951; Baxter & Sommerville, 2011).

To create that bridge, the book develops and applies the Human-Centric AI Governance Ecosystem Framework, which conceptualizes human-centric governance across three interdependent layers:

1. Macro (normative/regulatory): values, rights, and legal duties;
2. Meso (organizational/managerial): implementation decisions, oversight arrangements, and readiness; and
3. Micro (human experience/social legitimacy): trust, perceived safety, perceived dignity, and acceptance by those affected.

The framework provides a coherent way to interpret how ethical principles travel from regulations to organizations and, ultimately, to people.

Within this architecture, the book offers two complementary contributions. First, it clarifies how a human-centric approach is expressed and prioritized in the AI Act, not only as an abstract ideal but also as a regulatory orientation linked to protection of health, safety, fundamental rights, and public interests such as democracy and environmental protection.

The focus on future managers is particularly important because organizational adoption decisions increasingly depend on leaders capable of balancing innovation, ethical responsibility, stakeholder expectations, and technological transformation (Wodarski et al., 2025). These considerations are further reflected in broader discussions concerning AI-supported leadership, decision-making processes, human oversight, and the evolving role of humanoid robots in managerial environments (Skubis, 2025).

Third, the book introduces the Human-Centric Robot Acceptance Index (HCRAI), a multidimensional framework designed to assess managerial and organizational readiness for humanoid robot adoption in healthcare. Unlike traditional acceptance models that focus primarily on technological characteristics, the HCRAI integrates technical acceptance, ethical trust, governance assurance, managerial commitment, and patient safety perceptions.

Fourth, the book develops the Risk Gradient Model of Humanoid Robot Task Acceptance in Healthcare. The model demonstrates that acceptance is not uniform across healthcare functions but varies systematically according to perceived risk, responsibility, decision authority, and relational sensitivity.

Beyond bridging policy and practice, the book aims to support readers who work on governance, management, healthcare innovation, and responsible technology. It provides a conceptual structure for understanding why promising technologies remain stuck at the pilot stage, how oversight expectations shape adoption pathways, and why socio-technical alignment is often a stronger barrier than technical capability alone. The discussion is also relevant to broader processes of organizational transformation and innovation management in the era of digital transformation, where AI increasingly influences strategic decision-making, business models, and organizational capabilities (Kabus et al., 2026).

The discussion also contributes to broader debates concerning responsible AI, trustworthy AI, and human-centered innovation. These debates increasingly emphasize that successful technological transformation depends not only on technical performance but also on inclusion, human agency, ethical responsibility, and social legitimacy (OECD, 2019; World Health Organization, 2021).

The book is organized into four chapters. Chapter 1 examines the concept of human-centric AI within the European Union's Artificial Intelligence Act through qualitative content analysis of key concepts associated with human-centered governance. Chapter 2 moves from regulation to organizational practice by examining managerial readiness for humanoid robot adoption in healthcare through an empirical survey. Chapter 3 introduces the HCRAI as a multidimensional framework for assessing readiness for healthcare robot adoption. Chapter 4 develops the Risk Gradient Model of Humanoid Robot Task Acceptance, explaining how acceptance varies according to perceived risk, responsibility, and ethical sensitivity across different healthcare tasks.

Ultimately, the book argues that human-centric AI is not self-executing through regulation; it must be actively enacted through managerial choices and institutional design in ways that preserve dignity, agency, and trust.

REFERENCES

Baxter, G., & Sommerville, I. (2011). Socio-technical systems: From design methods to systems engineering. *Interacting with Computers*, *23*(1), 4–17. https://doi.org/10.1016/j.intcom.2010.07.003

Davis, F. D. (1989). Perceived usefulness, perceived ease of use, and user acceptance of information technology. *MIS Quarterly*, *13*(3), 319–340. https://doi.org/10.2307/249008

Dignum, V. (2019). *Responsible artificial intelligence: How to develop and use AI in a responsible way*. Springer. https://doi.org/10.1007/978-3-030-30371-6

Floridi, L., Cowls, J., Beltrametti, M., Chatila, R., Chazerand, P., Dignum, V., Luetge, C., Madelin, R., Pagallo, U., Rossi, F., Schafer, B., Valcke, P., & Vayena, E. (2018). AI4People-An ethical framework for a good AI society: Opportunities, risks, principles, and recommendations. *Minds and Machines*, *28*(4), 689–707. https://doi.org/10.1007/s11023-018-9482-5

Kabus, J., Antczak, J., Skubis, I., & Zajkowska, M. (2026). *Innovative business strategies: In the era of digital transformation*. Routledge.

OECD. (2019). *OECD AI principles overview*. Available at: https://oecd.ai/en/ai-principles

Rogers, E. (2003). *Diffusion of innovations*. Fifth edition. Free Press.

Shneiderman, B. (2020). Human-centered artificial intelligence: Reliable, safe and trustworthy. *International Journal of Human–Computer Interaction*, *36*(6), 495–504. https://doi.org/10.1080/10447318.2020.1741118

Skubis, I. (2025). Humanoid robots CEOs and leaders in project management: Decision-making, human oversight, team dynamics and ethics. *International Journal of Humanoid Robotics, 22*(6), 2550008. https://doi.org/10.1142/S0219843625500082

Skubis, I., Xerri, D., & Adamovic, M. (2026). *Human–AI collaboration in research: Practical applications, ethical frameworks, and future directions.* CRC Press.

Trist, E. L., & Bamforth, K. W. (1951). Some social and psychological consequences of the longwall method of coal-getting: An examination of the psychological situation and defences of a work group in relation to the social structure and technological content of the work system. *Human Relations*, *4*(1), 3–38. https://doi.org/10.1177/001872675100400101

Wodarski, K., Wodarska, J., & Skubis, I. (2025). *Professional Profile of a Top Manager in a Process and Project Organization. Scientific Papers of Silesian University of Technology. Organization and Management Series*, No. 237.

World Health Organization. (2021). *Ethics and governance of artificial intelligence for health*. World Health Organization.

Human-Centric Approach to Ethical AI Governance

1

The European Union's Artificial Intelligence Act

This chapter examines the concept of a human-centric approach in the European Union's Artificial Intelligence Act (AI Act), a landmark legal framework addressing the ethical governance of AI systems. Through qualitative content analysis, the study identifies and evaluates the occurrence and contextual significance of key terms – human-centric AI, human well-being, social and environmental well-being, user-friendliness, inclusivity, gender balance, and human dignity – within the Act's provisions. The findings highlight the Act's emphasis on aligning AI systems with societal values, fundamental rights, and ethical principles, ensuring inclusivity, autonomy, and public trust. Additionally, the analysis underlines the Act's focus on safeguarding public interests such as health, safety, democracy, and environmental sustainability while balancing innovation and regulation. By placing a strong emphasis on a human-centric approach and fostering accountability, transparency, and equity, the AI Act serves as a model for responsible AI governance. This research examines how the European Union's (EU) regulatory approach, as reflected in the AI Act, seeks to mitigate ethical risks and promote societal well-being through a human-centric legal framework.

DOI: 10.1201/9781042027200-2

1.1 ETHICAL AI GOVERNANCE

Ethical AI governance ensures alignment with human values, fundamental rights, and societal well-being. Recent scholarly work has emphasized the importance of a human-centric approach in AI governance. Choung et al. (2023) propose a multilevel framework involving governments, corporations, and citizens to ensure AI systems adhere to ethical standards and fundamental human values. Their study highlights the necessity of a collaborative governance structure to effectively translate ethical principles into practice.

Similarly, Tahaei et al. (2023) conduct a systematic literature review at the intersection of human-centered, ethical, and responsible AI, identifying key themes such as governance, fairness, and explainability. They advocate for expanding research to address potential unforeseen implications of AI, including areas like privacy, security, and human flourishing.

In the context of the EU, the AI Act, which entered into force on August 1, 2024, represents the world's first legal framework on AI. It aims to foster the development and uptake of safe and trustworthy AI systems across the EU, ensuring respect for fundamental rights, safety, and ethical principles by addressing the risks associated with powerful AI.

This chapter contributes to the ongoing discourse on AI ethics by analyzing the frequency and contextual significance of terms associated with a human-centric approach – such as human well-being, social and environmental well-being, user-friendliness, inclusivity, gender balance, and human dignity – within the AI Act. By examining these terms, the research demonstrated the Act's alignment with ethical AI principles and its implications for fostering trust, inclusivity, and societal well-being.

1.2 HUMAN-CENTRIC ARTIFICIAL INTELLIGENCE

Human-Centric Artificial Intelligence (HCAI) prioritizes ethical values, human rights, and societal well-being, addressing concerns over the rapid advancement of AI (Schmager et al., 2023). The EU emphasizes balancing technological growth with the protection of fundamental rights through a risk-based framework, as embodied in the AI Act.

HCAI prioritizes integrating high automation with robust human control to enhance human performance while ensuring reliability, safety, and trustworthiness (Shneiderman, 2020). Xu's (2019) tripartite framework identifies ethically aligned design, technology enhancement, and human factors design as core components, emphasizing the development of AI systems that are fair, comprehensible, and usable, supporting human agency and decision-making.

HCAI has been applied in various domains, showcasing its adaptability and impact. In smart cities, HCAI has facilitated privacy protection, ethical urban planning, and resident-centric services (Skubis, Wolniak, & Grebski, 2024; Dashkevych & Portnov, 2023; Pushkar et al., 2023; Bosco et al., 2024). In management, it has enhanced decision-making and organizational workflows through socio-technical systems and ethical AI tools (Dong et al., 2024; Skubis & Wodarski, 2023). Generative AI has benefited from HCAI in creative industries, aligning outputs with societal norms and user intent (Skubis, Wodarski, & Lütge, 2024; Riedl, 2019; Skubis & Kołodziejczyk, 2024; Chen et al., 2023). Tourism has seen HCAI applications that improve user engagement, trust, and personalized travel experiences (OECD, 2024; Skubis, Mesjasz-Lech, & Nowakowska-Grunt, 2024; Skubis, 2025; Huang et al., 2024). Healthcare has also leveraged HCAI to augment human expertise while maintaining ethical oversight (Andersen et al., 2023; Skubis, 2024; Turchi et al., 2024).

The incorporation of human-centered design (HCD) methodologies into AI development further strengthens the HCAI framework. HCD emphasizes iterative, stakeholder-driven processes to align technological solutions with diverse user needs and values (Dignum, 2019; Norman, 2005). By fostering empathy and inclusivity, HCD provides practical tools for addressing the ethical and societal implications of AI systems.

The AI Act establishes risk categories, ensuring stringent oversight of high-risk applications while fostering innovation. High-risk systems must adhere to strict transparency, safety, and accountability measures. These align with the EU's commitment to human dignity, autonomy, and anti-discrimination principles (Pirozzoli, 2024; van der Heijden, 2021; Aven & Renn, 2009).

The ethical and societal challenges of AI have prompted regulatory initiatives from governments, academia, and industry. Frameworks like the European Commission's Ethics Guidelines for Trustworthy AI emphasize transparency, accountability, inclusiveness, and a human-centric approach respecting human rights and societal well-being (AI-HLEG, 2019). Industry leaders contribute with frameworks such as IBM's AI Ethics Framework, which focuses on transparency, bias mitigation, and stakeholder participation (IBM, 2020), and Microsoft's Responsible AI Framework, which highlights inclusivity and fairness to address diverse user needs (Microsoft, 2024).

Despite significant progress, several challenges remain in the implementation of HCAI and its associated regulatory frameworks. The lack of a universally accepted definition of HCAI complicates efforts to standardize guidelines and promote international cooperation (Renz & Vladova, 2021). Additionally, the rapid pace of AI innovation often outstrips the development of regulatory mechanisms, creating gaps in oversight and accountability (Dwivedi et al., 2022). Effective AI regulation requires adaptability to emerging technologies and societal needs, collaboration among governments, academia, and industry, and inclusion of under-represented perspectives to enhance equity, trust, and acceptance across diverse contexts (Nicenboim et al., 2020).

1.3 ETHICAL DECISION-MAKING

Ethical decision-making models, such as those outlined by Rest (1986), provide a structured framework for addressing moral considerations in organizational contexts. When applied to AI, these models help organizations deal with ethical dilemmas, such as ensuring fairness, avoiding bias, and maintaining accountability (Floridi et al., 2020; Skubis, 2021). Moreover, the principles of fairness and accountability are closely tied to the design of ethical AI systems, as emphasized in research by Jobin et al. (2019). Integrating these models into AI strategies ensures that technologies respect human dignity and societal norms, fostering responsible AI deployment.

AI in management enhances routine decision-making, complementing human efforts in tasks like mergers and acquisitions while maintaining managerial control. Automation suits structured tasks, whereas augmentation excels in complex contexts requiring human intuition and creativity (Raisch & Krakowski, 2020; Skubis & Wodarski, 2023). AI also streamlines operations, fosters innovation, and shifts decision-making from principle-based to adaptive, data-driven models (Yano, 2017; Sundström, 2024; Skubis, 2024a; Schildt, 2017). However, this shift also brings challenges, including potential conflicts between inductive AI methods and traditional deductive management practices (Lambert & Sponem, 2012; Morales & Lambert, 2013). The integration of AI has redefined performance metrics and created new tensions in management control systems, emphasizing the need for rethinking management roles and systems (Fourcade & Healy, 2016).

While AI enhances structured decision-making by leveraging large datasets for efficiency, its application in semi-structured and unstructured decisions remains limited to providing recommendations and analytical insights rather than replacing human judgment entirely (Gümüsay et al., 2022). For instance, AI excels in tactical tasks like pricing and digital advertising but requires human oversight for strategic decisions, such as mergers or talent acquisition (Munir, 2019; Lahmann et al., 2018). AI's limitations in intuition, emotional intelligence, and creativity highlight the ongoing need for human involvement in ethical decision-making. Tasks requiring empathy, complex problem-solving, or interpersonal interactions depend on human managers, emphasizing the complementary strengths of humans and AI (Braga & Logan, 2017; Raisch & Krakowski, 2020; Skubis & Kołodziejczyk, 2024).

The EU's guidelines on trustworthy AI stress the importance of human agency and oversight throughout the AI lifecycle, including real-time monitoring, human validation, and operational constraints. These measures ensure accountability, transparency, and alignment with fundamental rights such as human dignity and societal well-being (AI-HLEG, 2019; White Paper, 2020; AI Act, 2024). EU policy also focuses on mitigating algorithmic bias and non-transparency by promoting fairness, accountability, and regular assessments to prevent discrimination and support responsible AI development and deployment (Skubis, 2024b).

1.4 METHODOLOGY

The methodology of this study focuses on a qualitative content analysis of the AI Act, a key regulatory framework proposed by the EU to establish harmonized rules for AI development, deployment, and governance. The analysis was conducted to explore how the concepts of human-centric AI, human well-being, social and environmental well-being, user-friendliness, inclusivity, gender balance, and human dignity are integrated into the AI Act's provisions. Furthermore, the notions of trustworthy AI, ethical AI, and safe AI were analyzed only when they appeared in conjunction with the primary terms listed above, allowing for a focused exploration of these terms in their specific contexts.

The AI Act (2024) was selected as the document for analysis due to its central role in shaping the ethical and regulatory landscape for AI within the EU. The Act provides a comprehensive legal framework designed to balance innovation with the protection of human rights, societal values, and public interests. As such, it serves as a critical text for understanding the EU's approach to the governance of AI technologies. The terms human-centric AI, human well-being, social and environmental well-being, user-friendliness, inclusivity, gender balance, and human dignity were selected as synonymous with a human-centric approach that prioritizes serving human beings.

These terms collectively represent the EU's emphasis on aligning AI development with societal values, fundamental rights, and equitable benefits. The research aimed to examine how frequently these terms appear within the text of the AI Act and to analyze the contexts in which they are employed. By quantifying their occurrences and interpreting their usage, the study sought to assess the extent to which the AI Act integrates and emphasizes the principles of a human-centric approach in its regulatory framework. This analysis provided insights into the alignment of the Act with ethical AI governance and its commitment to serving humanity.

This study focused solely on the AI Act, excluding supplementary documents and external sources. The analysis of trustworthy, ethical, and safe AI was limited to instances where these terms co-occurred with selected primary terms, as their standalone mentions were too frequent and broad. While the study centered on synonyms like human well-being, inclusivity, and human dignity, it did not capture all potential expressions of a human-centric approach, highlighting the complexity of interpreting human-centric values in regulatory texts.

1.5 RESEARCH OUTCOMES

Below, the research results outline the frequency and contextual significance of terms associated with a human-centric approach within the AI Act, providing details on how these principles are embedded in the regulatory framework to prioritize societal values, fundamental rights, and equitable outcomes.

Table 1.1 shows the occurrence and regulatory context of the term "human-centric and trustworthy AI" in the AI Act (p. 4, point 1), highlighting how the Regulation frames AI development in alignment with Union values and fundamental rights.

1.5.1 Human-Centric (and Trustworthy AI)

Analysis: The similar introduction is in "Chapter I General Provisions. *Article 1 Subject matter*" *point (1).* "Promote the uptake of human centric and trustworthy artificial intelligence (AI)": The Regulation explicitly prioritizes the adoption of human-centric AI, ensuring that technological progress aligns with societal needs and values. Human-centric AI is framed as both ethical and trustworthy, reflecting its alignment with human dignity, autonomy, and rights. It needs to be underlined that the term "human centric" appears in two forms – with a dash or without in the AI Act. In Table 1.1 and 1.5 of this chapter, it appears as two separate words. *"Protection of health, safety, fundamental rights"* will be discussed in the table of Chapter I General Provisions. **Implications:** This focus positions AI as a tool to support individuals and society rather than as an autonomous or unregulated force. It emphasizes

TABLE 1.1 Context 1

AI ACT	*CONTEXT*
Human centric and trustworthy AI p.4, point 1	"The purpose of this Regulation is to improve the functioning of the internal market by laying down a uniform legal framework (…) in accordance with Union values, to promote the uptake of **human centric** and ***trustworthy artificial intelligence (AI)*** while ensuring a high level of ***protection of health, safety, fundamental rights*** (...)"

TABLE 1.2 Context 2

AI ACT	*CONTEXT*
AI act p. 7, point 6	"Given the major impact that AI can have on society and the need to build trust, it is vital for AI and its regulatory framework to be developed in accordance with Union values (…). As a pre-requisite, AI should be a **human-centric** technology. It should serve as a tool for people, with the ultimate aim of increasing **human well-being** (…)"

human oversight and control over AI systems, particularly in high-impact areas like health, safety, and environmental protection.

Table 1.2 presents the reference in the AI Act (p. 7, point 6) that links human-centric AI to the promotion of human well-being, emphasizing AI as a tool for people and societal benefit.

1.5.2 Human-Centric and Human Well-Being

Analysis: "AI should be a human-centric technology": This positions human-centricity as a fundamental requirement for AI, emphasizing that systems must enhance human capabilities rather than replace them. AI is framed as a tool that operates under human control, ensuring that technology aligns with ethical principles and societal values. "With the ultimate aim of increasing human well-being": Human well-being is identified as the core outcome of AI deployment. This encompasses improving quality of life, public health, safety, and societal harmony. **Implications:** The Regulation prioritizes human-centric AI to enhance human capabilities, align with ethical values, and uphold democracy, dignity, and equality. By focusing on human autonomy, oversight, and

TABLE 1.3 Context 3

AI ACT	*CONTEXT*
AI act p. 7, point 8	"(...). By laying down those rules as well as measures in support of innovation with a particular focus on small and medium enterprises (SMEs), including startups, this Regulation supports the objective of promoting the European **human-centric approach to AI** and being a global leader in the development of secure, ***trustworthy and ethical AI*** as stated by the European Council, and it ensures the protection of ethical principles, as specifically requested by the European Parliament."

well-being, it ensures that AI systems improve quality of life and deliver equitable, long-term societal benefits.

Table 1.3 outlines the AI Act provision (p. 7, point 8) that promotes the European human-centric approach to AI alongside secure, trustworthy, and ethical development principles.

1.5.3 Human-Centric (Approach to AI), Trustworthy, and Ethical AI

Analysis: "Promoting the European human-centric approach to AI": The Regulation explicitly positions human-centricity as a cornerstone of its AI strategy, ensuring that AI systems serve societal needs and values rather than purely technical or economic goals.

"High level of protection of public interests, such as health and safety and the protection of fundamental rights"**:** A human-centric AI approach is tied to safeguarding critical public interests, including democracy, the rule of law, and environmental protection. This ensures that AI development respects human dignity and societal priorities.

" (…) development of secure, trustworthy and ethical AI" and "Ensuring the protection of ethical principles": The explicit connection between human-centric AI and secure, trustworthy, and ethical guidelines reinforces a development framework that prioritizes human oversight, accountability, and trustworthiness.

Implications: A human-centric approach ensures AI aligns with societal values, protects public interests like democracy and safety, and prioritizes ethical principles such as accountability and trustworthiness, fostering responsible innovation and public trust.

TABLE 1.4 Context 4

AI ACT	*CONTEXT*
AI act p. 27, point 27	"(...) In those guidelines, the AI HLEG developed seven non-binding ethical principles for AI which are intended to help ensure that **AI is trustworthy and ethically sound.** (...) those guidelines contribute to the design of a coherent, trustworthy and **human-centric AI**, in line with the Charter and with the values on which the Union is founded. According to the guidelines of the AI HLEG, human agency and oversight means that AI systems are developed and used as a tool that serves people, respects **human dignity and personal autonomy**, and that is functioning in a way that can be appropriately controlled and overseen by humans." (.....) **Social and environmental well-being** means that AI systems are developed and used in a sustainable and environmentally friendly manner as well as in a way to **benefit all human beings** (...)."

Table 1.4 summarizes the AI Act reference (p. 27, point 27) where human-centric AI is connected to social and environmental well-being, ensuring that AI benefits all human beings.

1.5.4 Human-Centric AI; Social and Environmental Well-Being; To Benefit All Human Beings

Analysis: "Trustworthy and human-centric AI, in line with the Charter and with the values on which the Union is founded": Human-centric AI is emphasized as a cornerstone of the EU's approach, linking AI development to principles of human agency, oversight, and respect for autonomy.

"Social and environmental well-being" is defined as the development and use of AI systems in ways that are sustainable, environmentally friendly, and **beneficial to all human beings.** It also emphasizes the importance of monitoring and assessing long-term impacts on individuals, society, and democracy.

Implications: By prioritizing human oversight and agency, the EU ensures that AI systems uphold values like dignity, autonomy, and fairness. This framework mitigates risks such as loss of control, bias, or dehumanization in AI applications.

TABLE 1.5 Context 5

AI ACT	*CONTEXT*
CHAPTER I GENERAL PROVISIONS *Article 1* *Subject matter* p. 160, point 1	"The purpose of this Regulation is to improve the functioning of the internal market and promote the uptake of **human-centric and trustworthy artificial intelligence (AI)**, while ensuring **a high level of protection of health, safety, fundamental rights** enshrined in the Charter of Fundamental Rights (...)."

Table 1.5 displays the statement in the AI Act (Chapter I, Article 1, p. 160, point 1) reinforcing the objective of promoting human-centric and trustworthy AI while safeguarding fundamental rights.

1.5.5 Human-Centric (and Trustworthy) AI

Analysis: "Promote the uptake of human-centric and trustworthy artificial intelligence (AI)": This term appears also in point 1 (Table 1.1) and point 176 (Table 1.6). The Regulation explicitly identifies human-centric AI as a core objective, emphasizing its alignment with human values and societal needs. Human-centricity ensures AI systems serve as tools that enhance human capabilities and autonomy while minimizing risks. "Ensuring a high level of protection of health, safety, fundamental rights": This clause reinforces the protective role of human-centric AI, which prioritizes safeguarding individual well-being and societal interests over purely technical or commercial objectives. "In accordance with Union values, to promote... fundamental rights as enshrined in the Charter of Fundamental Rights of the European Union": The explicit mention of the Charter ensures that AI regulation is grounded in principles like democracy, equality, and the rule of law. Human-centricity is deeply tied to protecting these rights. **Implications:** The Regulation's focus on human-centric AI emphasizes aligning technology with fundamental rights and societal values, safeguarding dignity, autonomy, and well-being. Grounded in the Charter of Fundamental Rights, it ensures that AI systems enhance human capabilities while protecting against risks like discrimination, privacy loss, and threats to democracy.

Table 1.6 highlights the AI Act's recital 176, which reaffirms the goal of promoting human-centric and trustworthy AI while protecting health, safety, democracy, and the environment.

TABLE 1.6 Context 6

AI ACT	*CONTEXT*
(176)	Since the objective of this Regulation, namely to improve the functioning of the internal market and promoting the uptake of ***human centric*** **and trustworthy AI**, while ensuring a **high level of protection of health, safety, fundamental rights** enshrined in the Charter, including democracy, the rule of law and environmental protection against harmful effects of AI systems in the Union and supporting innovation (…). In accordance with **the principle of proportionality as set out in that Article,** this Regulation does not go beyond what is necessary in order to achieve that objective.

1.5.6 Human-Centric (and Trustworthy) AI

Analysis: "Promoting the uptake of human centric and trustworthy AI": This expression is mentioned in Table 1.1 and Table 1.5. When it comes to the term "human centric" itself, in this article 176, it emerges without a dash as two separate words. The Regulation highlights human-centric AI as essential for achieving societal goals, ensuring that AI systems respect human dignity, autonomy, and fundamental rights. "Ensuring a high level of protection of health, safety, fundamental rights": This term is mentioned in Table 1.1 and Table 1.5. Human-centricity is tied to safeguarding public interests, including health, safety, democracy, and environmental protection. These are aligned with the values enshrined in the Charter of Fundamental Rights. "In accordance with the principle of proportionality... does not go beyond what is necessary": The Regulation adheres to principles of proportionality and subsidiarity, ensuring that human-centric AI governance is effective without imposing unnecessary restrictions. **Implications:** The Regulation emphasizes human-centric AI as essential for protecting dignity, autonomy, and fundamental rights, aligning with public interests like health, safety, democracy, and environmental protection. By adhering to proportionality and subsidiarity, it balances effective oversight with fostering innovation, ensuring that AI development mitigates risks such as discrimination and privacy breaches while prioritizing societal well-being.

Table 1.7 presents the AI Act reference (p. 117, point 131) describing the need for a publicly accessible, transparent, and user-friendly database of AI systems.

TABLE 1.7 Context 7

AI ACT	*CONTEXT*
p. 117, point 131	"(...). This section of the database should be publicly accessible, free of charge, the information should be easily navigable, understandable and machine-readable. The database should also be **user-friendly,** for example by providing search functionalities, (...)."

1.5.7 User-Friendly

Analysis: This passage emphasizes the importance of making AI-related information accessible and comprehensible to diverse stakeholders, with a focus on transparency and usability. "The database should also be user-friendly, for example by providing search functionalities, including through keywords": The term "user-friendly" is applied to the design of a database for high-risk AI systems, emphasizing ease of use and accessibility for the general public and stakeholders.

"Information should be easily navigable, understandable, and machine-readable": The database's design aims to ensure that users can efficiently access and interpret critical information about high-risk AI systems. "Publicly accessible, free of charge": Ensuring free public access to the database reflects a commitment to inclusivity and transparency, enabling citizens, organizations, and regulators to engage with AI-related information. **Implications:** A user-friendly, publicly accessible database ensures transparency and inclusivity by allowing all stakeholders, including non-experts, to easily access and interpret information about high-risk AI systems. This fosters trust, accountability, and equitable engagement while supporting informed decision-making and oversight.

Table 1.8 shows the AI Act provision (Chapter VIII, Article 71, p. 344, point 4) requiring the EU database for high-risk AI systems to be accessible in a user-friendly manner.

TABLE 1.8 Context 8

AI ACT	*CONTEXT*
Chapter VIII EU Database For High-Risk AI Systems *Article 71 EU database for high-risk AI systems listed in Annex III* p. 344, point 4	"(...) the information contained in the EU database registered in accordance with Article 49 shall be accessible and publicly available in a **user-friendly** manner."

1.5.8 User-Friendly

Analysis: "The information contained in the EU database... shall be accessible and publicly available in a user-friendly manner": The Regulation mandates that the EU database for high-risk AI systems be designed to facilitate easy access and use by the general public and stakeholders. "Easily navigable and machine-readable": The database must allow users to locate and interpret information effortlessly, regardless of their technical expertise. "Accessible only to market surveillance authorities and the Commission... unless consent is given for public access": While user-friendliness is prioritized, certain sensitive information is restricted to authorities to protect privacy and proprietary details, unless providers agree to public access. **Implications:** The Regulation ensures a user-friendly database for high-risk AI systems, promoting inclusivity and

TABLE 1.9 Context 9

AI ACT	*CONTEXT*
(165), p. 149	"The development of AI systems other than high-risk AI systems in accordance with the requirements of this Regulation may lead to a larger uptake of ***ethical and trustworthy AI*** in the Union. (...) Providers and, as appropriate, deployers of all AI systems, high-risk or not, and AI models should also be encouraged to apply on a voluntary basis additional requirements related, for example, to the elements of the Union's Ethics Guidelines for Trustworthy AI, environmental sustainability, AI literacy measures, **inclusive and diverse design** and development of AI systems, including attention to vulnerable persons and accessibility to persons with disability, stakeholders' participation with the involvement, as appropriate, of relevant stakeholders such as business and civil society organisations, academia, research organisations, trade unions and consumer protection organisation in the design and development of AI systems, and ***diversity of the development teams, including*** **gender balance**. To ensure that the voluntary codes of conduct are effective, they should be based on clear objectives and key performance indicators to measure the achievement of those objectives. They should also be ***developed in an*** **inclusive way,** as appropriate, with the involvement of relevant stakeholders such as business and civil society organisations, academia, research organisations, trade unions and consumer protection organisation."

trust by allowing easy access to information for all stakeholders. While prioritizing transparency, it balances accessibility with confidentiality, safeguarding privacy and proprietary details, and reflecting the EU's commitment to ethical and secure AI governance.

Table 1.9 summarizes the AI Act's recital 165 (p. 149), which encourages inclusive and diverse AI design, stakeholder participation, and gender balance in development teams.

1.5.9 Inclusive AI, Gender Balance

Analysis: "Inclusive and diverse design and development of AI systems, including attention to vulnerable persons and accessibility to persons with disability": The Regulation explicitly promotes inclusive AI design, emphasizing the need to consider the needs of vulnerable groups and ensure accessibility for persons with disabilities. "To ensure that the voluntary codes of conduct are effective, they should be developed in an inclusive way": Inclusivity is also extended to the development of governance mechanisms, ensuring that ethical guidelines and codes of conduct reflect diverse stakeholder input. "Diversity of the development teams, including gender balance": The Regulation emphasizes the importance of diverse development teams, recognizing that inclusivity at the design stage can reduce biases in AI systems. "Encouraged to apply on a voluntary basis additional requirements related, for example, to... inclusive and diverse design": The Regulation supports voluntary adherence to inclusive design principles for all AI systems, even those not classified as high-risk. "The Commission may develop initiatives (…) to facilitate... interoperability of different types of data": By addressing technical barriers to data sharing and collaboration, the Regulation supports inclusivity across sectors and borders, ensuring that AI development benefits a broad range of stakeholders. **Implications:** The Regulation emphasizes inclusive AI design by addressing

TABLE 1.10 Context 10

AI ACT	*CONTEXT*
Chapter X Codes Of Conduct And Guidelines. Article 95. Codes of conduct for voluntary application of specific requirements	2. (d) facilitating an **inclusive and diverse design** of AI systems, including through the establishment of **inclusive and diverse development teams** and the promotion of stakeholders' participation in that process (…).

the needs of vulnerable groups, ensuring accessibility, and promoting diverse development teams. By fostering stakeholder participation and supporting voluntary adherence to inclusivity principles, it reduces biases, enhances fairness, and improves societal impact. Additionally, sectoral initiatives to facilitate data interoperability promote inclusivity across contexts, ensuring that AI systems benefit all stakeholders and reflect diverse societal needs.

Table 1.10 presents the AI Act's Article 95 provision on voluntary codes of conduct, reinforcing the importance of inclusive and diverse AI system design.

1.5.10 Inclusive AI

Analysis: Repetition of what was mentioned in point (165) – Table 1.9.

Table 1.11 shows the AI Act recital 27 reference to human dignity and personal autonomy in the context of human agency and oversight in AI systems.

1.5.11 Human Dignity

Analysis: "Respects human dignity and personal autonomy": AI systems are framed as tools that serve people, preserving their autonomy and safeguarding their inherent dignity. "Appropriately controlled and overseen by humans": This reinforces the principle that AI should augment human capabilities without undermining individual control or independence. **Implications:** These provisions ensure that AI systems operate ethically, avoiding scenarios where AI might diminish individual rights or subject humans to unchecked automated decision-making.

Table 1.12 outlines the AI Act recital 28, which prohibits manipulative and exploitative AI practices that violate human dignity and other fundamental rights.

TABLE 1.11 Context 11

AI ACT	*CONTEXT*
(27)	(...). According to the guidelines of the AI HLEG, human agency and oversight means that AI systems are developed and used as a tool that serves people, respects **human dignity** and personal autonomy, and that is functioning in a way that can be appropriately controlled and overseen by humans.

TABLE 1.12 Context 12

AI ACT	*CONTEXT*
(28)	"Aside from the many beneficial uses of AI, that technology can also be misused and provide novel and powerful tools for manipulative, exploitative and social control practices. Such practices are particularly harmful and abusive and should be prohibited because they contradict Union values of respect for **human dignity,** freedom, equality, democracy and the rule of law and fundamental rights enshrined in the Charter, including the right to non-discrimination, to data protection and to privacy and the rights of the child."

1.5.12 Human Dignity

Analysis: "AI can also be misused... for manipulative, exploitative and social control practices": The excerpt identifies the potential harms of AI, particularly its capacity to enable practices that undermine individual autonomy and dignity. "Such practices... should be prohibited because they contradict Union values of respect for human dignity, freedom, equality, democracy, and the rule of law": The passage ties respect for human dignity to broader Union values, including equality and democratic governance. Practices that undermine dignity are explicitly framed as violations of these core principles. "Fundamental rights enshrined in the Charter, including the right to non-discrimination, to data protection and to privacy and the rights of the child": The reference to the Charter emphasizes the EU's legal framework for protecting individuals against abuses, ensuring that AI respects rights such as privacy, non-discrimination, and protections for vulnerable groups like children. **Implications:** The EU explicitly prohibits exploitative and manipulative AI practices to protect individual autonomy, dignity, and fundamental rights. By aligning AI regulation with core Union values – such as democracy, equality, and the rule of law – and the rights enshrined in the Charter, including privacy and non-discrimination, the EU ensures ethical AI development that safeguards societal well-being and provides special protections for vulnerable groups, including children.

Table 1.13 presents the AI Act recital 48 (p. 44), where human dignity is identified as a key criterion in classifying AI systems as high-risk.

1.5.13 Human Dignity

Analysis: "The extent of the adverse impact... on fundamental rights": The Regulation establishes that the potential impact of AI on fundamental rights,

TABLE 1.13 Context 13

AI ACT	*CONTEXT*
(48), p. 44	"The extent of the adverse impact caused by the AI system on the fundamental rights protected by the Charter is of particular relevance when classifying an AI system as high risk. Those rights include the right to **human dignity**, respect for private and family life, protection of personal data, freedom of expression and information, (…)."

TABLE 1.14 Context 14

AI ACT	*CONTEXT*
(58), p. 55	"(….) AI systems are used for determining whether such benefits and services should be granted, denied, reduced, revoked or reclaimed by authorities, (…) and may infringe their fundamental rights, such as the right to social protection, non-discrimination, **human dignity** or an effective remedy and should therefore be classified as high-risk."

particularly human dignity, is a critical factor in classifying AI systems as high-risk. This ensures that systems with significant societal or individual implications receive stricter oversight. "Rights include the right to human dignity, respect for private and family life, protection of personal data, freedom of expression and information": Human dignity is placed at the forefront of the rights to be protected, alongside privacy and freedom, ensuring that AI development adheres to ethical standards and respects individual autonomy. **Implications:** By classifying AI systems with adverse impacts on human dignity as high-risk, the Regulation enforces stricter accountability and safeguards. This ensures that AI systems are designed and deployed in ways that protect and uphold fundamental rights, emphasizing the EU's commitment to ethical AI governance that prioritizes individual dignity and societal trust.

Table 1.14 shows the AI Act recital 58 (p. 55), which recognizes that certain AI systems affecting social benefits and services may infringe human dignity and must be considered high-risk.

1.5.14 Human Dignity

Analysis: "AI systems... may have a significant impact on persons' livelihood": The passage identifies the critical role of AI in decisions regarding benefits and services, which directly affect individuals' well-being and societal inclusion. "May infringe their fundamental rights... such as human dignity": The potential for AI systems to undermine fundamental rights, including human dignity, is explicitly acknowledged. This highlights the ethical risks of automated decision-making in areas essential to individuals' livelihoods.

"Should therefore be classified as high-risk": AI systems with such far-reaching implications are designated as high-risk, requiring stringent oversight and accountability to prevent harm and protect rights.

Implications: By classifying these systems as high-risk, the Regulation ensures that AI technologies used in critical social protection decisions adhere to strict ethical and legal standards. This safeguards fundamental rights, including human dignity, by preventing misuse and ensuring fairness and accountability in decisions that deeply impact individuals' lives and well-being.

1.6 CONCLUSIONS

This research highlights the AI Act's strong commitment to embedding a human-centric approach within its regulatory framework. By analyzing terms such as human-centric AI, human well-being, social and environmental well-being, user-friendliness, inclusivity, gender balance, and human dignity, the study reveals how the Act seeks to align AI development and deployment with the core values of the EU. These values – grounded in democracy, human rights, and societal well-being – serve as a foundation for ensuring that AI systems function as tools to support human agency, autonomy, and dignity.

In the analysis of the AI Act tables, the term "human-centric" appears in two distinct forms. It was used twice as two separate words, "human centric," and four times as a compound word, "human-centric." This variation in usage suggests both flexibility in phrasing and an evolving preference for the compound form in formal contexts within the legislative framework. "Human well-being" was referenced twice under two expressions: as "human well-being" and "to benefit all human beings," underlining its importance in aligning AI with societal benefits. "User-friendly" occurred twice, emphasizing accessibility and usability in AI systems. The phrase "social and environmental well-being" was used once, reflecting the interconnected societal and environmental priorities in AI governance. The word "inclusive" appeared four times in the following expressions: "inclusive and diverse design and development of AI systems," "They should also be developed in an inclusive way," "facilitating an inclusive and diverse design of AI systems," and "establishment of inclusive and diverse development teams." "Gender balance" was mentioned once, underscoring the commitment to diversity and equitable AI development. Lastly, "human dignity" was noted four times, emphasizing its foundational role in ensuring respect for individual rights and autonomy within the regulatory framework. These frequencies demonstrate the Act's focus on aligning AI systems with ethical and human-centric principles.

The appearance of these terms within the AI Act, particularly in conjunction with concepts like trustworthy AI, ethical AI, and safe AI, highlights a deliberate effort to create a regulatory environment that fosters trust and inclusivity while mitigating risks such as discrimination, bias, and environmental harm. The Act's emphasis on sustainability and equitable benefits further demonstrates its holistic approach to addressing the societal and environmental impacts of AI technologies. While the selected terms provide a clear lens for examining the human-centric focus of the AI Act, it is important to acknowledge that a human-centric approach can be expressed in various ways beyond these specific terms. This research, therefore, represents a focused but not exhaustive exploration of the language and principles embedded in the Act. The findings suggest that the AI Act serves as a robust framework for guiding ethical AI governance, offering a model for balancing innovation with the protection of human dignity and societal values.

Future research could expand upon these insights by analyzing supplementary documents or exploring how these principles are implemented in practice across different AI systems and use cases. By doing so, it would be possible to evaluate the Act's real-world impact in fostering a trustworthy, inclusive, and sustainable AI ecosystem.

While this chapter examined how the AI Act incorporates a human-centric approach at the regulatory level, the realization of these principles depends on organizational actors who interpret and implement them. In high-stakes domains such as healthcare, implementation decisions involve not only compliance but also trust-building, workflow redesign, and continuous human oversight. The next chapter, therefore, moves from regulatory language toward the organizational and managerial level and analyzes how future managers evaluate humanoid robots in healthcare through perceived usefulness, perceived ease of use, ethical trust, and socio-technical readiness.

REFERENCES

AI Act (Artificial Intelligence Act). (2024).
AI-HLEG. (2019). *Ethics guidelines for trustworthy AI.* European Commission.

Andersen, T. O., Nunes, F., Wilcox, L., Coiera, E., & Rogers, Y. (2023). Introduction to the special issue on human-centred AI in healthcare: Challenges appearing in the wild. *ACM Transactions on Computer-Human Interaction, 30*(2), Article 25. https://doi.org/10.1145/3589961

Aven, T., & Renn, O. (2009). On risk defined as an event where the outcome is uncertain. *Journal of Risk Research, 12*(1), 1–11. https://doi.org/10.1080/13669870802488883

Bosco, G., Riccardi, V., Sciarrone, A., D'Amore, R., & Visvizi, A. (2024). AI-driven innovation in smart city governance: Achieving human-centric and sustainable outcomes. *Transforming Government: People, Process and Policy, 20*(1), 98–123. https://doi.org/10.1108/TG-04-2024-0096

Braga, A., & Logan, R. K. (2017). The emperor of strong AI has no clothes: Limits to artificial intelligence. *Information, 8*, 156. https://doi.org/10.3390/info8040156

Chen, X. A., Burke, J., & Du, R. (2023). Next steps for human-centered generative AI: A technical perspective. https://doi.org/10.48550/arXiv.2306.15774

Choung, H., David, P., & Seberger, J. S. (2023). A multilevel framework for AI governance. https://doi.org/10.48550/arXiv.2307.03198

Dashkevych, O., & Portnov, B. A. (2023). Human-centric, sustainability-driven approach to ranking smart cities worldwide. *Technology in Society, 74*, 102296. https://doi.org/10.1016/j.techsoc.2023.102296

Dignum, V. (2019). *Responsible artificial intelligence: How to develop and use AI in a responsible way*. Springer.

Dong, M., Bonnefon, J. F., & Rahwan, I. (2024). Toward human-centered AI management: Methodological challenges and future directions. *Technovation, 131*(C), 102953. https://doi.org/10.1016/j.technovation.2024.102953

Dwivedi, Y. K., Hughes, L., Kar, A. K., et al. (2022). Climate change and COP26: Are digital technologies and information management part of the problem or the solution? An editorial reflection and call to action. *International Journal of Information Management, 63*, 1–39. https://doi.org/10.1016/j.ijinfomgt.2021.102456

Floridi, L., Cowls, J., King, T. C., & Taddeo, M. (2020). How to design AI for social good: Seven essential factors. *Science and Engineering Ethics, 26*(3), 1771–1796. https://doi.org/10.1007/s11948-020-00213-5

Fourcade, M., & Healy, K. (2016). Seeing like a market. *Socio-Economic Review, 15*(1), 9–29.

Gümüsay, A., Bohné, T., & Davenport, T. (2022). AI and the future of management decision-making. *Management and Business Review, 3*(3), 1–19. www.researchgate.net/publication/363404836_AI_and_the_Future_of_Management_Decision-Making

Huang, A., Ozturk, A. B., Zhang, T., de la Mora Velasco, E., & Haney, A. (2024). Unpacking AI for hospitality and tourism services: Exploring the role of perceived enjoyment on future use intentions. *International Journal of Hospitality Management, 119*. www.sciencedirect.com/science/article/abs/pii/S0278431924000057?via%3Dihub

IBM. (2020). *AI ethics framework*.

Jobin, A., Ienca, M., & Vayena, E. (2019). The global landscape of AI ethics guidelines. *Nature Machine Intelligence, 1*, 389–399.

Lahmann, M., Keiser, P., & Stierli, A. (2018). AI will transform project management. *Are You Ready?* www.pwc.ch/en/insights/risk/transformation-assurance-ai-will-transform-project-management-are-you-ready.html

Lambert, C., & Sponem, S. (2012). Roles, authority, and involvement of the management accounting function: A multiple case-study perspective. *European Accounting Review, 21*(3), 565–589. https://doi.org/10.1080/09638180.2011.629415

Microsoft. (2024). *RAI transparency report.*

Morales, J., & Lambert, C. (2013). Dirty work and the construction of identity: An ethnographic study of management accounting practices. *Accounting, Organizations and Society, 38*(3), 228–244.

Munir, M. (2019). How artificial intelligence can help project managers. *Global Journal of Management and Business Research, 19*(1), 1–8.

Nicenboim, I., Giaccardi, E., Søndergaard, M. L. J., et al. (2020). More-than-human design and AI: In conversation with agents. *Companion publication of the 2020 ACM designing interactive systems conference*, 397–400. https://doi.org/10.1145/3393914.3395912

Norman, D. A. (2005). Human-centered design considered harmful. *Interactions, 12*(4), 14–19. https://doi.org/10.1145/1070960.1070976

OECD. (2024). *Artificial intelligence and tourism: G7/OECD policy paper*. OECD Tourism Papers, Paris. http://dx.doi.org/10.1787/3f9a4d8d-en

Pirozzoli, A. (2024). The human-centric perspective in the regulation of AI. *European Papers, 9*(1), 105–116.

Pushkar, T., Serogina, D., Matvieieva, N., Sobolieva, H., & Zhovtyak, H. (2023). HCI approach to shaping smart city development strategies. In O. Arsenyeva, T. Romanova, M. Sukhonos, I. Biletskyi, & Y. Tsegelnyk (Eds.), *Smart technologies in urban engineering* (Vol. 808). Springer https://doi.org/10.1007/978-3-031-46877-3_3

Raisch, S., & Krakowski, S. (2020). Artificial intelligence and management: The automation-augmentation paradox. *Academy of Management Review, 46*(1). https://doi.org/10.5465/amr.2018.0072

Renz, A., & Vladova, G. (2021). Reinvigorating the discourse on human-centered artificial intelligence in educational technologies. *Technology Innovation Management Review, 11*(5), 5–16. https://doi.org/10.22215/timreview/1438

Rest, J. R. (1986). *Moral development: Advances in research and theory.* Praeger.

Riedl, M. O. (2019). Human-centered artificial intelligence and machine learning. *Human Behavior and Emerging Technologies, 1*(1), 33–36. https://doi.org/10.1002/hbe2.117

Schildt, H. (2017). Big data and organizational design: The brave new world of algorithmic management and computer-augmented transparency. *Innovation, 19*(1), 23–30.

Schmager, S., Pappas, I., & Vassilakopoulou, P. (2023). Defining human-centered AI: A comprehensive review of HCAI literature. www.researchgate.net/publication/373019807_Defining_Human-Centered_AI_A_Comprehensive_Review_of_HCAI_Literature

Shneiderman, B. (2020). Human-centered artificial intelligence: Reliable, safe & trustworthy. *International Journal of Human–Computer Interaction, 36*(6), 495–504. https://doi.org/10.1080/10447318.2020.1741118

Skubis, I. (2021). Językoznawstwo jako bezpieczna dyscyplina dla badań nad sztuczną inteligencją. In B. Fischer, A. Pązik, & M. Świerczyński (Eds.), *Prawo sztucznej inteligencji i nowych technologii* (pp. 169–181). Wolters Kluwer.

Skubis, I. (2024). Ética, terminología, opiniones y el mercado de SexTech: Un análisis multidisciplinario sobre los robots sexuales. *Wydawnictwo Politechniki Śląskiej*. ISBN: 978-83-7880-957-9

Skubis, I. (2024a). Seksroboty – Zarządzanie Etyką i Zarządzanie Innowacjami w Branży Sextech. *Management and Quality*, *6*(3), 211–232.

Skubis, I. (2024b). The EU guidelines on roboethics and ethics of sex robots. In Ch. Lütge, A. Kriebitz, R. Max, & C. Corrigan (Eds.), *The Elgar companion to applied AI ethics* (pp. 397–409). Edward Elgar Publishing.

Skubis, I. (2025). Exploring the potential and perceptions of social robots in tourism and hospitality: Insights from industry executives and technology evaluation. *International Journal of Social Robotics, 17*, 59–72. https://doi.org/10.1007/s12369-024-01197-z

Skubis, I., & Kołodziejczyk, D. (2024). *Human vs ChatGPT – Language of advertising in beauty products advertisements*. Taylor and Francis.

Skubis, I., Mesjasz-Lech, A., & Nowakowska-Grunt, J. (2024). Humanoid robots in tourism and hospitality – Exploring managerial, ethical, and societal challenges. *Applied Sciences*, *14*(24), 11823. https://doi.org/10.3390/app142411823

Skubis, I., & Wodarski, K. (2023). Humanoid robots in managerial positions – Decision-making process and human oversight. *Scientific Papers of Silesian University of Technology*, *189*, 573–596. http://dx.doi.org/10.29119/1641-3466.2023.189.36

Skubis, I., Wodarski, K., & Lütge, Ch. (2024). Human-ChatGPT interaction: Prompt analysis on the basis of sex robots' topic – linguistic, social and ethical considerations of generative AI. *Linguistic and Philosophical Investigations*, *23*(1), 2467–2485.

Skubis, I., Wolniak, R., & Grebski, W. (2024). AI and human-centric approach in smart cities management: Case studies from Silesian and Lesser Poland Voivodships. *Sustainability*, *16*(18), 8279. https://doi.org/10.3390/su16188279

Sundström, A. (2024). AI in management control: Emergent forms, practices, and infrastructures. *Critical Perspectives on Accounting, 99*, 102701. https://doi.org/10.1016/j.cpa.2023.102701

Tahaei, M., Constantinides, M., Quercia, D., & Muller, M. (2023). A systematic literature review of human-centered, ethical, and responsible AI. https://doi.org/10.48550/arXiv.2302.05284

Turchi, T., Prencipe, G., Malizia, A., Filogna, S., Latrofa, F., & Sgandurra, G. (2024). Pathways to democratized healthcare: Envisioning human-centered AI-as-a-service for customized diagnosis and rehabilitation. *Artificial Intelligence in Medicine, 151*. https://doi.org/10.1016/j.artmed.2024.102850

van der Heijden, J. (2021). Risk as an approach to regulatory governance: An evidence synthesis and research agenda. *Sage Open, 11*(3). https://doi.org/10.1177/21582440211032202

White Paper on Artificial Intelligence. (2020). *A European approach to excellence and trust.*

Xu, W. (2019). Toward human-centered AI: A perspective from human-computer interaction. *Interactions*, *26*(4), 42–46. https://doi.org/10.1145/3328485

Yano, K. (2017). How artificial intelligence will change HR. *People Strategy, 40*(1), 42–47.

Human-Centric Adoption of Humanoid Robots in Healthcare

2

Trust, Ethics, and Managerial Readiness

Building on the regulatory foundations of human-centric AI governance discussed in Chapter 1, this chapter examines whether human-centric principles are likely to be enacted in practice through managerial adoption decisions. By integrating technology acceptance, diffusion, socio-technical alignment, and responsible AI governance, the chapter investigates how trust, oversight, usability, and perceived legitimacy shape readiness to deploy humanoid robots in healthcare contexts.

2.1 AI IN HEALTHCARE

Healthcare systems are under intensifying pressure to deliver safer, more efficient, and more patient-centered services amid workforce shortages and rising demand. Social and humanoid robots have emerged as a visible strand of this

 DOI: 10.1201/9781042027200-3

digital transformation, promising gains in logistics, triage, rehabilitation, and routine clinical tasks; yet real-world uptake remains uneven and often stalls at the pilot stage due to concerns about usability, workflow fit, ethics, and trust (Greenhalgh et al., 2004; Berwick, 2003). Understanding managerial acceptance is therefore essential: managers translate technological potential into investment, implementation, and scale-up decisions that shape whether robots complement human work or remain isolated experiments (Holden & Karsh, 2010).

To explain acceptance, we base the study in the Technology Acceptance Model (TAM), where Perceived Usefulness (PU) and Perceived Ease of Use (PEOU) drive attitudes and behavioral intention (Davis, 1989; Davis et al., 1989). Extensions of TAM underline the role of social influence, job relevance, output quality, and facilitating conditions, factors that are salient in complex healthcare settings (Venkatesh & Davis, 2000; Venkatesh & Bala, 2008; Legris et al., 2003).

Prior healthcare studies consistently show that both PU and PEOU predict clinicians' willingness to adopt digital tools such as electronic health records (EHRs), telemedicine, and m-health, while organizational support and trust moderate these relationships (Yarbrough & Smith, 2007; Maillet et al., 2015; Rahimi et al., 2018; Tubaishat, 2017). Recent work also indicates that younger cohorts and future leaders evaluate AI-enabled systems, including humanoid robots, through the joint lens of expected benefits and human oversight, linking TAM constructs to managerial intention (Skubis, 2025b; Wirtz et al., 2018).

Because acceptance unfolds over time, we complement TAM with Diffusion of Innovation (DoI), which traces movement from knowledge and persuasion to decision, implementation, and confirmation (Rogers, 1962, 2003). In healthcare, diffusion hinges not only on perceived advantage but also on compatibility with professional norms, trialability, and observability, alongside robust stakeholder engagement (Greenhalgh et al., 2004; Berwick, 2003; Cresswell & Sheikh, 2013). We further adopt a Socio-Technical Systems (STS) perspective to capture how technical changes (robot capabilities, interoperability) must co-evolve with social systems (roles, skills, culture) to avoid misalignment that undermines performance and acceptance (Trist & Bamforth, 1951; Pasmore, 1988; Trist & Murray, 1993; Baxter & Sommerville, 2011).

Finally, acceptance of healthcare robots is inseparable from ethics and trust. The EU's Ethics Guidelines for Trustworthy AI articulate seven requirements, human agency and oversight, robustness and safety, privacy and data governance, transparency, diversity and fairness, societal well-being, and accountability, that increasingly underpin managerial governance and the AI Act's risk-based approach (European Commission, 2019, 2021; Floridi et al., 2018).

Trust develops from initial cues (representation, explainability, trialability, peer reviews) to continuous performance (usability, reliability, collaboration, security, interpretability), while unresolved concerns about job displacement or goal misalignment can erode confidence (Siau & Wang, 2018). A human-centric management stance, prioritizing human dignity, agency, and responsible leadership, thus provides a normative compass for integrating robots in ways that preserve empathy and accountability (Friedman & Hendry, 2019; Maak & Pless, 2006; Voegtlin et al., 2012; Skubis, 2025c).

Against this backdrop, our study examines how familiarity, ethics and trust, organizational readiness, and TAM constructs shape managerial support for humanoid robots in healthcare. Using a survey of management students (future managers), we map questionnaire sections to TAM (PU, PEOU), DoI stages, STS alignment, and responsible AI governance to identify where acceptance is facilitated or blocked, and to derive actionable implications for leaders planning robot integration.

2.2 TECHNOLOGY ACCEPTANCE MODEL (TAM)

The TAM, introduced by Fred Davis (1989), is one of the most influential theoretical frameworks in management and information systems research. It explains how users come to accept and use new technologies, emphasizing two primary determinants: PU and PEOU. According to Davis (1989), PU refers to "the degree to which a person believes that using a particular system would enhance his or her job performance," while PEOU denotes "the degree to which a person believes that using a particular system would be free of effort." These constructs influence attitudes toward technology, which in turn affect behavioral intention and ultimately actual system use (Davis, 1989; Davis et al., 1989).

Since its introduction, TAM has become a cornerstone of managerial decision-making research in contexts involving technological innovation. It provides a parsimonious and empirically validated framework for understanding how individuals and organizations evaluate technological change (Venkatesh & Davis, 2000; Venkatesh & Bala, 2008). The model has been particularly valuable in management studies because it links perceived performance improvement and operational feasibility, two essential managerial considerations, directly to adoption intentions (Legris et al., 2003).

In healthcare management, TAM has been extensively applied to assess the acceptance of digital innovations such as electronic health records (Holden & Karsh, 2010), telemedicine systems (Yarbrough & Smith, 2007), and mobile health applications (Rahimi et al., 2018). These studies consistently demonstrate that both PU and PEOU significantly predict healthcare professionals' willingness to adopt new technologies. For instance, Tubaishat (2017) found that PU and PEOU explained a substantial proportion of nurses' behavioral intentions to use electronic health record systems. Similarly, Maillet et al. (2015) observed that PU and PEOU influenced clinicians' adoption of telemonitoring technologies, though trust and organizational support moderated these relationships.

In healthcare organizations, the managerial interpretation of TAM extends beyond user behavior to encompass organizational readiness and strategic implementation (Holden & Karsh, 2010; Alalwan et al., 2017). Within this managerial framework, PU represents the expected strategic or operational benefit, that is, whether humanoid robots are viewed as improving quality of care, workflow efficiency, and service delivery. PEOU reflects the feasibility of integration, the degree to which managers believe such systems can be implemented with minimal disruption, training, and resource constraints.

The application of TAM to humanoid robots in healthcare management allows researchers to assess how managerial stakeholders evaluate these technologies not only as innovations but as organizational tools that can support decision-making, improve patient care, and optimize administrative processes (Wirtz et al. 2018). In recent work, Skubis (2025a) demonstrated that acceptance of AI and humanoid robots in leadership and management among Generation Z students depends heavily on PU and human oversight. Similarly, Skubis (2025a) found that managerial perception of social and humanoid robots in hospitality was influenced by both TAM-related constructs and ethical trust. The model thus provides a conceptual foundation for interpreting managerial readiness toward humanoid robots in healthcare, linking perceived benefits and usability with ethical and organizational trust.

In this study, the questions about "usefulness" and "ease of use" of the questionnaire operationalize PU and PEOU, respectively, while the questions about "support and readiness" capture behavioral intention, which corresponds to managerial support for implementation.

From a management standpoint, TAM thus provides a robust theoretical lens to interpret innovation acceptance, perceived performance enhancement, and integration readiness. If managers or future healthcare leaders perceive humanoid robots as useful and easy to integrate, they are more likely to advocate for their implementation within healthcare systems.

Conversely, if robots are perceived as difficult to use or offering marginal improvements, managerial resistance and ethical hesitation may increase. This underlines TAM's enduring value in strategic innovation management and in understanding the human and organizational determinants of digital transformation in healthcare.

2.3 DIFFUSION OF INNOVATION THEORY (ROGERS, 2003)

The DoI theory by Rogers (1962, 2003) explains how technological innovations spread through social systems over time. It identifies five stages: knowledge, persuasion, decision, implementation, and confirmation; and five perceived attributes of innovations: relative advantage, compatibility, complexity, trialability, and observability.

DoI theory has been successfully applied to explain adoption of medical technologies and digital tools in hospitals (Greenhalgh et al., 2004; Berwick, 2003). In this study, respondents' familiarity corresponds to the *Knowledge* stage, their ethical trust and perceived safety to *Persuasion*, and managerial support and resource allocation to the *Decision* and *Implementation* stages.

Building on Rogers' diffusion framework, recent research emphasizes that social and ethical legitimacy, not just technological advantage, determines adoption in healthcare (Cresswell & Sheikh, 2013; Scarbrough & Kyratsis, 2022). Skubis and Wodarski (2023) highlight similar dynamics in managerial decision-making about AI-driven leadership, adoption progresses only when technological innovation is socially and ethically compatible with existing human values and management norms.

2.4 SOCIO-TECHNICAL SYSTEMS THEORY (TRIST & BAMFORTH, 1951)

The STS approach, developed by Trist and Bamforth (1951) at the Tavistock Institute, conceptualizes organizations as comprising interdependent social and technical subsystems. Fox's (1995) discussion of the STS approach emphasizes the need to integrate both the technical and social dimensions of organizations to achieve optimal performance. He argues that these two systems are interdependent, what benefits one may not suit the other, thus requiring a balance through joint optimization.

Technological innovation requires simultaneous adaptation in social structures, processes, and relationships to maintain system equilibrium (Trist & Murray, 1993; Pasmore, 1988). In healthcare, STS theory can be used to study digital transformation and robotics integration. Implementing humanoid robots affects not only technical workflows but also staff roles, communication patterns, and the ethical climate of care (Skubis et al., 2024) The results of answers on management and implementation in this study highlighting staff resistance, ethical concerns, and investment barriers align with STS predictions about socio-technical misalignment.

2.5 TRUST AND RESPONSIBLE MANAGEMENT FRAMEWORKS AND HUMAN-CENTRIC MANAGEMENT PERSPECTIVE

The Ethics Guidelines for Trustworthy AI (European Commission, 2019) established seven key requirements for responsible AI: *human agency and oversight*, *technical robustness and safety*, *privacy and data governance*, *transparency*, *diversity and fairness*, *societal well-being*, and *accountability*. These guidelines, and later the EU AI Act, have become central to managerial governance of AI systems across sectors (Coeckelbergh, 2025; Floridi et al., 2018).

Initial and continuous trust in AI-enabled humanoid robots hinge on specific technology features and governance choices. For initial trust, representation and perception matter: humanlike or familiar embodiments (e.g., humanoids, robot dogs) can ease emotional connection, yet sci-fi-shaped fears of "runaway AI" depress trust; positive user reviews, transparency, explainability, and opportunities to try before adopting (trialability) all raise early trust (Siau & Wang, 2018).

Continuous trust then depends on day-to-day usability, reliability, smooth human–AI collaboration/communication, sociability, robust security/privacy, and ongoing interpretability; unresolved worries about job displacement and goal misalignment erode trust unless mitigated by retraining and clear governance (Siau & Wang, 2018).

Extending this to sensitive social-robot domains, ethical trust must also guard human dignity, consent, agency, and societal impacts, areas the EU has highlighted but where domain-specific guidance (e.g., for intimate or highly relational robots) remains underdeveloped (Coeckelbergh, 2020; Skubis, 2024).

Within healthcare, responsible management involves ensuring human oversight, safeguarding patient rights, and embedding transparency in decision-support systems (European Commission, 2021). Ethical governance has become a managerial competency, linking trust with strategic legitimacy. In line with this, managerial attitudes toward AI technologies depend not only on perceived efficiency but also on ethical transparency and regulatory compliance Skubis (2025b). In healthcare, responsible management translates these principles into practice via human oversight, patient-rights safeguards, and transparent decision support, linking ethical governance to strategic legitimacy and managerial acceptance (European Commission, 2019; European Commission, 2021). Consistent with our findings, managerial attitudes toward AI depend not only on perceived efficiency but also on ethical transparency and regulatory compliance, situating adoption at the intersection of TAM(PU/PEOU), DoI (persuasion/decision), and trustworthy, human-aligned AI.

The Human-Centric Management Perspective situates AI and robotics within responsible and sustainable management theories that prioritize human well-being, agency, and trust. Drawing from responsible leadership theory (Maak & Pless, 2006; Voegtlin et al., 2012) and value-sensitive design principles (Friedman & Hendry, 2019), it asserts that technology should *serve people*, not replace them.

In healthcare, this means ensuring that humanoid robots complement rather than substitute human empathy and decision-making. The EU's vision of "human-centric AI" reinforces this ethos, promoting innovation that supports social trust, accountability, and ethical reflection.

2.6 METHODOLOGY

2.6.1 Research Design and Ethical Approval

This study adopted a quantitative survey design to examine perceptions, ethical attitudes, and managerial readiness toward social and humanoid robots in healthcare. The research aimed to explore the extent to which TAM variables, PU and PEOU, as well as trust, ethical awareness, and innovation diffusion stages influence future managers' acceptance of AI-enabled humanoid robots in healthcare contexts.

Prior to data collection, the study underwent an ethical review process and received a favorable opinion from the institutional Research Ethics Committee. The approval confirmed that the study met the standards of research integrity, confidentiality, and voluntary participation in accordance with institutional and European ethical guidelines for human research. Participants were provided with a Participant Information Form and a Participant Communication Letter, which explained the purpose, procedures, risks, and rights associated with the research. Participation was entirely voluntary, and participants were informed of their right to withdraw at any stage without providing a reason.

All collected data were anonymous and used solely for academic purposes. The ethical review emphasized compliance with the EU General Data Protection Regulation (GDPR), the European Code of Conduct for Research Integrity, and the Ethics Guidelines for Trustworthy AI (European Commission, 2019), particularly in relation to privacy, informed consent, and safeguarding of participants' dignity.

2.6.2 Participants and Sampling

The target population consisted of respondents enrolled in management-related programs, representing future and early-career managers as well as prospective decision-makers. Given the predominance of Master's-level students, some participants already possess professional or managerial experience, providing insights from both educational and workplace perspectives. The experience comes from employment, internships, or alternance (work-study/apprenticeship) contracts, allowing them to combine academic learning with practical organizational experience. Consequently, the sample reflects not only future managerial perspectives but also insights informed by workplace exposure. This population was selected because of its relevance to managerial innovation adoption and its position at the intersection of academic learning and emerging professional practice.

A total of 527 valid responses were collected through an online survey distributed via academic channels. The sample was balanced by gender (51% female, 49% male) and primarily composed of Management Master's-level students (96%), with the dominant age group between 23 and 26 years. This group represents early-career professionals, digital natives, who are likely to influence managerial decision-making processes in healthcare digitalization and AI usage.

2.6.3 Instrumentation

The research instrument consisted of a structured questionnaire composed of 30 closed-ended questions divided into six sections:

1. Demographics: age, gender, and academic level.
2. Familiarity: exposure to AI, robotics education, and interaction with humanoid robots.
3. Ethics and Trust: participants' ethical concerns, trust levels, and attitudes toward human oversight.
4. Management and Implementation: perceived challenges, integration support, and resource allocation preferences.

5. Technological Acceptance: PU and PEOU, based on TAM constructs.
6. Future Outlook: expectations regarding humanoid robots in healthcare and interest in further learning.

Each item was rated using five- or four-point Likert-type scales, depending on the construct measured.

2.6.4 Data Collection Procedure and Data Analysis

Data were collected online over a four-week period. Participants received a link to the questionnaire along with the Participant Information Form and Communication Letter. Respondents were assured that their answers would remain confidential, that data would be stored securely, and that results would be reported only in aggregate form.

The questionnaire was administered through the Qualtrics platform and distributed via the Sona System to ensure reliable participant recruitment and data management. Descriptive statistics were used to summarize demographic variables and response distributions across questionnaire sections. Where relevant, the results were interpreted through the following theories:

- TAM (Davis, 1989; Venkatesh & Davis, 2000);
- DoI (Rogers, 2003);
- STS theory (Trist & Bamforth, 1951; Pasmore, 1988);
- Trust and Responsible Management Frameworks (European Commission, 2019; Floridi et al., 2018).

These frameworks were used to contextualize managerial attitudes toward the adoption of humanoid robots in healthcare, considering technological feasibility, social acceptance, ethical governance, and alignment with human-centric management principles (Maak & Pless, 2006; Voegtlin et al., 2012; Friedman & Hendry, 2019).

2.6.5 Ethical Considerations

The study fully adhered to ethical research principles as defined by the European Code of Conduct for Research Integrity and institutional Research Integrity Policy. Ethical safeguards included:

- Informed consent prior to participation;
- Voluntary participation and right to withdraw;

- Confidentiality and anonymity of all responses;
- Compliance with GDPR for data protection;
- Ethical oversight approval granted by the institutional Research Ethics Committee.

These procedures ensured that the study respected participants' autonomy and privacy while upholding the integrity and transparency required in research on emerging technologies and AI ethics.

2.6.6 Research Questions and Hypotheses

The research questions and hypotheses for the study were as follows:

Research Questions

1. How do PU and PEOU affect managerial readiness for robot integration in healthcare?
2. How do ethical trust and oversight influence acceptance?
3. Does prior familiarity with robotics increase readiness for implementation?
4. What are the main barriers perceived by managers regarding robot integration?

Hypotheses

- **H1:** Higher *PU* of humanoid robots increases *managerial support* for integration in healthcare management.
- **H2:** Greater *PEOU* positively influences *PU*.
- **H3:** *Ethical concerns* (e.g., data privacy, loss of human touch) negatively correlate with *managerial acceptance*.
- **H4:** Higher *trust* in humanoid robots positively predicts *willingness to allocate resources* for implementation.
- **H5:** Greater *familiarity* with robotics (knowledge and exposure) increases *organizational readiness*.

2.6.7 Research Outcomes

2.6.7.1 Demographic Information

A total of 527 valid responses were recorded for the demographic section of the questionnaire, encompassing age, gender, and academic level. The sample represents primarily young, academically active individuals enrolled in management-related programs, corresponding to the study's focus on future healthcare managers and decision-makers. Although the respondents were predominantly enrolled in MA studies, many individuals in French higher education participate in alternance (work-study/apprenticeship) programs or maintain professional employment while studying. Therefore, the findings capture both academic perceptions and experiences derived from real organizational environments.

For the item "What is your age group?", the largest segment of respondents belonged to the 23–26 years old category (76%), followed by 18–22 years old (18%), 27–30 years old (4%), 31–35 years old (1%), and only a few respondents aged 36–40 (0.5%) or 41–45 years old (0.5%).

Age groups were numerically coded from 1 (18–22) to 6 (41–45) for analytical purposes. The mean coded value was 1.91 (SD = 0.60), indicating that respondents were concentrated in the youngest age categories. The distribution confirms a predominantly young and relatively homogeneous cohort, representing individuals at an early stage of their professional and managerial development, many of whom are likely to influence future decisions regarding innovation, digital transformation, and AI adoption.

For "What is your gender?", responses were well-balanced, with female respondents representing 51% and male respondents 48%. A small proportion – 1% preferred not to disclose their gender. Such balance enhances the robustness of the findings, ensuring that perspectives are not disproportionately shaped by a single gender group.

In terms of educational attainment ("What is your academic level?"), the vast majority of respondents were enrolled in Master's (MA) programs (96%), while 3% were enrolled in undergraduate (BA) programs and 1% in doctoral (PhD) programs. Many Master's-level participants may also have been engaged in professional activities through employment, internships, or alternance (work-study) arrangements, reflecting a combination of academic and workplace experience. This distribution aligns with the study's methodological focus on future managerial and administrative professionals: a population positioned between academic learning and professional practice.

Overall, the demographic structure demonstrates a young, highly educated, and gender-balanced cohort, predominantly composed of individuals enrolled in Master's-level programs and aged between 23 and 26 years. The low variability in both age and educational level indicates that the sample is demographically consistent, capturing the perspectives of individuals at an early stage of their professional and managerial development. Many respondents may also possess practical workplace experience through employment, internships, or alternance (work-study) arrangements, providing insights that extend beyond purely academic perspectives.

From a management and innovation perspective, such a population is particularly relevant to the TAM and the DoI framework. Younger, well-educated individuals, often classified as digital natives, tend to exhibit higher openness toward technological adoption, perceive new tools as useful and easy to use, and are more responsive to innovation-driven organizational strategies. Their views provide valuable information about managerial readiness and ethical acceptance of humanoid and social robots in healthcare.

2.6.7.2 General Information and Familiarity

2.6.7.2.1 Exposure to AI and Robotics Education
Among 527 respondents who addressed the question on prior AI or robotics coursework, 64% reported having taken at least one relevant course, whereas 36% indicated no prior coursework in these fields. From a management education perspective, this indicates that a majority of future healthcare managers possess at least foundational literacy in AI and robotics, an important precondition for informed decision-making regarding digital transformation. Such exposure aligns with the Knowledge stage of the DoI model, which highlights awareness and understanding as the first drivers of adoption.

2.6.7.2.2 Interaction Experience with Humanoid or Social Robots
Regarding prior interaction with humanoid or social robots, 9% of respondents reported encounters in healthcare settings, 33% in other environments such as retail or hospitality, 43% had been exposed to such robots only through media, and 15% indicated no familiarity with them.

This distribution suggests that while real-life interaction with healthcare robots remains limited, conceptual familiarity, often derived from media and non-healthcare settings, is widespread. Within the DoI framework, this stage represents knowledge acquisition through observation, which supports subsequent Persuasion and Decision stages of innovation diffusion.

2.6.7.2.3 Familiarity with Humanoid and Social Robots in Healthcare
For the question assessing familiarity levels, 37% reported being not familiar at all, 42% were slightly familiar, 19% were moderately familiar, and only 2% were very familiar with humanoid robots in healthcare.

This result highlights a gap between general awareness and domain-specific understanding. From a managerial standpoint, this gap may hinder evidence-based decision-making about robot adoption. Therefore, managerial training programs should focus on bridging conceptual familiarity with operational knowledge.

2.6.7.2.4 Academic Discussion of AI and Robots in Healthcare
Responses to whether AI and robots in healthcare had been studied or discussed during participants' programs reveal that 5% had studied the topic in-depth,

39% had discussed it briefly, 45% had not yet studied but expressed interest, and 11% had no interest in doing so.

These findings reinforce the Knowledge–Persuasion transition in the DoI model: the majority are aware of AI in healthcare and open to learning more, but few have engaged deeply with the topic. This educational readiness forms a foundational base for shaping ethical, managerial, and technical attitudes toward robot adoption.

Overall, the results indicate that the respondent group exhibits high theoretical awareness but limited practical familiarity with humanoid and social robots in healthcare contexts. Two-thirds have completed AI-related coursework, yet direct interaction with robots, especially in clinical settings, remains rare. These outcomes reflect the early diffusion phase of robotics in healthcare education and management.

From a management and innovation perspective, this stage corresponds to organizational knowledge accumulation, where leaders understand the existence and potential of technology but lack deep operational insight. Strategically, educational institutions can support this emerging interest through experiential learning modules, interdisciplinary projects, and ethical reflection workshops that bridge AI theory and healthcare practice.

2.6.7.3 Ethics, Trust, and Acceptance

2.6.7.3.1 Trust in Humanoid Robots for Care Provision

Levels of trust in humanoid robots providing care in hospitals or elderly settings varied, with 6% expressing full trust, 30% indicating somewhat trust, 36% remaining neutral, 24% reporting somewhat distrust, and 4% expressing full distrust. This distribution suggests that while respondents are not overtly resistant, there remains substantial hesitancy linked to reliability and empathy concerns.

From a management standpoint, this moderate trust aligns with the Persuasion stage in the *DoI* model, where awareness is established but conviction is still forming. Managers interpreting these results would note that trust must be cultivated through transparency, reliability demonstrations, and ethical assurance before large-scale implementation.

2.6.7.3.2 Ethical Concerns

Respondents most frequently identified loss of human touch in patient care (39%) as their primary ethical concern, followed by bias in AI decision-making (24%), data privacy and security (18%), dependency on robots over human caregivers (10%), and unemployment risks (7%). Only 2% reported no ethical concerns, viewing robots as beneficial.

In management terms, these data underline the critical role of ethical leadership and responsible innovation frameworks. Respondents' focus on human connection and bias mitigation indicates that ethical alignment, communication, and trust mechanisms are essential determinants of managerial acceptance and organizational legitimacy.

2.6.7.3.3 Willingness to Be Treated by a Robot

Willingness to be treated by a humanoid robot for a non-critical consultation showed that 12% were completely willing, 44% agreed under human supervision, 19% were neutral, 18% hesitant, and 7% would refuse. This finding directly supports the Trustworthy AI principle that humans should remain "in the loop," ensuring accountability and ethical safety.

From a managerial adoption perspective, this conditional acceptance reveals that future healthcare managers are willing to engage with robot-assisted care as long as oversight and accountability are preserved. Such attitudes indicate readiness for hybrid human–robot collaboration models rather than full automation.

2.6.7.3.4 Importance of Human Oversight

Regarding the importance of human oversight, 25% rated it extremely important, 28% very important, 22% moderately important, 21% slightly important, and 4% not important at all.

These results align with the EU's Trustworthy AI framework (2019), particularly principles of human agency, oversight, and accountability. Managers appear to value human control as a necessary safeguard, confirming that trust and oversight are interdependent in healthcare robotics acceptance.

Overall, findings illustrate that trust in humanoid robots is moderate but dependent on ethical assurances and human supervision. Ethical concerns, particularly around human empathy, bias, and privacy, reflect an emphasis on responsible management over technological enthusiasm. Respondents support adoption in a controlled, supervised, and ethically guided framework, resonating with both *STS* and *Responsible AI* governance.

From a managerial perspective, the implications are clear:

1. Ethical governance and communication strategies are prerequisites for trust building.
2. Transparency and human oversight mechanisms must accompany deployment to maintain legitimacy.
3. Training in ethical AI management should be integrated into healthcare leadership curricula to bridge the gap between technological capability and human-centered responsibility.

2.6.7.4 Management and Implementation

2.6.7.4.1 Support for Integration of Humanoid Robots

Support for the integration of humanoid robots in hospitals and healthcare management showed that 11% expressed *strong support*, 41% *somewhat support*, 29% were *neutral*, 15% *somewhat oppose*, and 4% *strongly oppose*.

From a managerial perspective, this suggests an openness to technological adoption under structured and ethically governed conditions. Within the *DoI* framework, this pattern corresponds to the Decision stage, where individuals begin evaluating practical feasibility and institutional readiness rather than abstract ethical principles.

2.6.7.4.2 Perceived Implementation Challenges

Respondents were allowed to select multiple challenges. The top-ranked obstacle was lack of public trust and acceptance (71%), followed by ethical and regulatory concerns (56%), resistance from medical staff (52%), high costs and investment (50%), and technological limitations (25%). These results reflect a perceived tension between technological potential and socio-organizational readiness.

Interpreted through STS theory, the data highlight that successful robot integration depends on aligning technical feasibility with social dynamics within healthcare institutions. Public perception and staff readiness are as critical as financial and technological capabilities, reinforcing the managerial need for strategic communication, change management, and stakeholder inclusion.

2.6.7.4.3 Preferred Roles for Humanoid Robots

In terms of healthcare roles, 49% of respondents favored administrative tasks, 25% preferred assistance with physical tasks, 13% identified social companionship, 9% selected medical advice or monitoring, and 4% believed robots should not be used at all. This result aligns with a gradual adoption strategy consistent with innovation diffusion theory, wherein organizations initially deploy robots in support functions that minimize ethical risk and staff resistance.

For management, this reflects a cautious but strategic approach to technology integration, prioritizing efficiency and staff support over direct patient interaction.

2.6.7.4.4 Resource Allocation Intentions

Regarding managerial willingness to allocate resources for robot integration, 9% would do so without hesitation, 57% only in specific areas, 18% were neutral, 12% hesitant, and 4% would not support such investments. This pattern shows conditional managerial support, reflecting cost–benefit awareness and selective implementation preferences.

This conditional attitude emphasizes responsible managerial behavior and the influence of perceived organizational alignment, key elements of STS, and responsible AI frameworks. Managers appear willing to endorse robotic solutions when they clearly demonstrate value, cost efficiency, and ethical oversight.

Overall, results demonstrate that managerial readiness for humanoid robot adoption is cautious but constructive. Respondents largely endorse selective, purpose-driven implementation that complements existing human roles rather than replaces them. The main managerial takeaways include:

1. Selective Integration: Early adoption should prioritize administrative and logistical functions, aligning with resource efficiency goals.
2. Ethical and Organizational Readiness: Lack of trust, regulatory ambiguity, and staff resistance must be addressed through transparent governance and training.
3. Investment Strategy: Managers show pragmatic budgeting behavior: allocating resources where return on investment (ROI), ethical compliance, and workforce acceptance converge.

These findings corroborate the Decision–Implementation stage of the *DoI* process and the alignment principle of *STS theory*. From a management standpoint, they suggest a transition from ethical deliberation toward strategic, evidence-based adoption, emphasizing both responsibility and operational feasibility.

2.6.7.5 Technological Acceptance

2.6.7.5.1 Perceived Usefulness (PU)

For the item assessing the PU of humanoid robots in improving healthcare services, 12% considered them not useful at all, 24% slightly useful, 34% moderately useful, 20% very useful, and 10% extremely useful. This distribution indicates moderate PU: respondents acknowledge potential benefits in efficiency, accuracy, and administrative relief, yet remain uncertain about the robots' impact on quality of care or patient well-being.

In TAM terms, this reflects partial alignment with the *PU* construct, showing openness to technological benefits but suggesting that empirical evidence and use-case visibility are necessary to solidify managerial conviction.

2.6.7.5.2 Perceived Ease of Use (PEOU)

Regarding ease of adaptation for hospital staff, 11% described it as extremely difficult, 47% as somewhat difficult, 28% as neutral, 13% as somewhat easy, and 1% as extremely easy.

This pattern underlines one of the main managerial challenges identified in TAM research: even if usefulness is acknowledged, low ease of use reduces adoption likelihood. Training, user-centered design, and supportive leadership will be critical to improving PEOU and thus behavioral intention to adopt.

2.6.7.5.3 Perceived Patient Safety and Acceptance

Half of the respondents (50%) believe that patients would feel more vulnerable when assisted by humanoid robots rather than human nurses, while 25% expect no difference, 7% think patients would feel safer, and 19% were unsure. These responses suggest that perceived patient vulnerability is a major concern.

From a management viewpoint, this result demonstrates that trust and human oversight remain decisive external variables influencing TAM constructs. Even when robots are perceived as useful, managerial support will depend on perceived patient safety and social acceptability – key determinants of responsible innovation.

2.6.7.5.4 Personal Treatment Preferences

Personal preferences for treatment showed that 28% preferred always being treated by a human, 45% were mostly open to robots with human oversight, 18% were neutral, 9% preferred mostly robot-led care, and 1% would always choose a robot.

This response pattern reinforces findings from earlier sections: technological acceptance is conditional on human supervision. Managers thus face a dual task, to maintain patient confidence while advancing automation efficiency, a balancing act central to the Human-Centric Management Perspective.

Results reflect partial acceptance of humanoid robots as useful but not yet easy to implement or fully trusted. Respondents perceive tangible benefits in operational support yet doubt adaptability, user-friendliness, and patient comfort. This configuration mirrors classic TAM dynamics, where PU outweighs PEOU, limiting behavioral intention.

From a management theory perspective:

1. TAM Integration: PU is moderately positive, but low PEOU and safety concerns constrain managerial adoption.
2. DoI Reinforcement: Respondents appear in the *Persuasion–Decision* stages: recognizing innovation potential but not fully convinced of operational feasibility.
3. STS Implication: Technological systems must be co-designed with human users to ensure workflow and social harmony.

2.6.7.6 Future Outlook

2.6.7.6.1 Beliefs about Error Reduction

Views on whether humanoid robots could enhance patient care by reducing medical errors were mixed: 6% strongly disagreed, 24% somewhat disagreed, 35% were neutral, 29% somewhat agreed, and 6% strongly agreed. These responses reveal cautious optimism – a moderate belief in robots' potential to improve accuracy but persistent doubt about their clinical reliability.

From a managerial standpoint, this result suggests a recognition of the *theoretical efficiency benefits* of automation while acknowledging uncertainty about practical reliability, ethical accountability, and human–machine coordination. It highlights the need for empirical validation, transparent error accountability, and trust calibration before large-scale clinical deployment.

2.6.7.6.2 Forecast for the Next Decade

In projecting the future of humanoid robots in healthcare, 20% predicted they would become common and widely accepted, 51% expected use with public hesitation, 25% foresaw limited use due to ethical or social concerns, and 4% believed they would fail to integrate. This pattern indicates a moderate expectation of conditional adoption, reflecting technological presence coupled with societal caution.

This finding aligns with the Confirmation stage of the *DoI* model, where participants envision selective implementation contingent on public trust and ethical maturity. From a management perspective, respondents anticipate a hybrid model where robots complement rather than replace human workers, echoing trends observed in early smart hospital initiatives.

2.6.7.6.3 Interest in Further Learning

Regarding interest in further learning about the management and ethical considerations of AI and robots, 9% were definitely interested, 36% rather interested, 34% were neutral, 14% rather not interested, and 7% definitely not interested. This distribution demonstrates moderate-to-high interest in educational engagement.

This interest suggests that respondents recognize the strategic importance of AI governance literacy and ethical competence as essential elements of leadership and decision-making in digital healthcare. It further supports integrating courses on *AI ethics, policy, and responsible management* into academic curricula and executive training programs.

Responses across the questions about a future outlook indicate a measured but forward-looking outlook among emerging managers. Although respondents perceived considerable potential benefits associated with humanoid robots, they also identified significant challenges concerning ethics, trust, and societal readiness. The prevailing attitude is "conditional optimism": confidence in technological innovation when supported by responsible management and ethical oversight. This aligns with a human-centric vision of healthcare digitalization, emphasizing balance between efficiency, empathy, and accountability.

From a managerial and theoretical perspective:

1. DoI: Respondents predict a sustained *early adoption phase*, with acceptance dependent on visible benefits and ethical assurance.
2. Responsible AI Governance: Ethical readiness and transparency will determine whether robots move from experimental to mainstream roles.
3. Human-Centric Management: Continuous professional education in AI ethics and governance is viewed as key to sustaining trust-based integration.

2.6.8 Discussion of Findings

RQ1. Perceived Usefulness (PU) and Ease of Use (PEOU) → Managerial Readiness

Respondents generally recognize the potential usefulness of humanoid robots in healthcare management, particularly for administrative and logistical tasks. Most participants associate robotic systems with efficiency, reliability, and workload reduction but remain cautious about their ease of implementation. The data reveal that a majority view robots as potentially useful, yet almost half expect their integration to be difficult, citing interoperability challenges and the need for extensive staff training. This pattern is consistent with the TAM (Davis, 1989; Venkatesh & Davis, 2000): PU may encourage intention to adopt, but low PEOU constrains readiness.

Managerial support is strongest for low-risk, back-office functions: 49% favor administrative uses and 25% physical assistance, reflecting early-phase adoption dynamics where perceived risk is minimal and benefits observable. In practical terms, managers appear willing to advocate for robotic integration only when implementation is expected to complement, not disrupt, human workflows. Thus, readiness is conditional on balancing technological potential with perceived usability and operational stability.

RQ2. Ethical Trust and Oversight → Acceptance

Trust clearly mediates managerial acceptance. While a portion of respondents express moderate confidence in robot-assisted care, 44% support their use only under human supervision, reflecting an endorsement of hybrid human–machine collaboration. Ethical trust is closely linked to transparency, accountability, and the preservation of human oversight – core components of the EU's *Ethics Guidelines for Trustworthy AI* (European Commission, 2019).

Key concerns center on the loss of human touch (39%), bias in AI decision-making (24%), and data privacy or security (18%). These findings confirm that ethical apprehensions remain major barriers to adoption. The insistence on human control mirrors the "human-in-the-loop" and "human-on-the-loop" principles, underscoring that oversight mechanisms are essential for legitimizing robotic decision support in healthcare (Floridi et al., 2018; Coeckelbergh, 2020). Hence, ethical governance and transparent communication strategies must precede full-scale deployment to sustain trust among both professionals and patients.

RQ3: Familiarity → Readiness

Approximately 64% of respondents reported completing at least one course related to AI or robotics, suggesting solid theoretical literacy. However, only 9% had direct interaction with humanoid robots in healthcare and 33% in other settings, while 43% were familiar only through media exposure. This gap between educational awareness and practical experience indicates that familiarity remains largely conceptual rather than experiential.

From the perspective of the DoI theory (Rogers, 2003), participants occupy the Knowledge and Persuasion stages: they understand the potential of robotics but have not yet formed strong behavioral intentions to adopt. Increasing exposure through pilot demonstrations, simulation training, and interdisciplinary education could accelerate progression toward the Decision and Implementation stages. In management education, this implies the need for experiential learning that bridges theoretical knowledge with ethical and operational realities of AI integration.

RQ4. Main Perceived Barriers

Respondents most frequently identified lack of public trust and acceptance (71%), followed by ethical and regulatory uncertainty (56%), staff resistance (52%), and high investment costs (50%) as principal challenges to robot adoption. Only one in four respondents mentioned technical limitations (25%) as a major concern, suggesting that socio-organizational rather than purely technical factors drive hesitation.

This configuration aligns closely with STS theory (Trist & Bamforth, 1951; Pasmore, 1988), which posits that technological innovations succeed only when social and technical subsystems are jointly optimized. In this context, the misalignment between innovation potential and social readiness, particularly concerning staff engagement, ethical clarity, and cost justification, appears as the central barrier to adoption. Managerial strategies that prioritize communication, co-design with staff, and transparent ethical oversight could help restore balance between these interdependent systems.

2.6.9 Conclusions

This study examined the managerial acceptance of humanoid and social robots in healthcare within the context of the TAM, DoI, STS theory, and responsible/human-centric AI governance. Across 527 respondents, the findings portray conditional optimism: robots are perceived as moderately useful (PU ≈ 2.94/5) yet not easy to implement (PEOU low; a majority anticipate difficulties), and acceptance is explicitly contingent on human oversight. Trust levels are cautious (neutral–somewhat trusting), and perceived patient vulnerability remains a salient concern. Together, the patterns indicate a readiness to adopt humanoid robots in low-risk, supportive roles first (administration, logistics), accompanied by selective resource allocation and staged deployment.

From a TAM perspective, the adoption ceiling is currently set by PEOU and trust/ethics rather than usefulness alone. Managers (and future managers) acknowledge potential efficiency and quality benefits, but foresee workflow disruption, training needs, and interoperability burdens that depress ease-of-use expectations and, consequently, behavioral intention. In DoI terms, the cohort sits between persuasion and decision: knowledge and interest are high (notably, 64% completed at least one AI/robotics course), but conviction hinges on credible demonstrations (trialability/observability) and on social legitimacy. The STS view clarifies why. The main barriers respondents cite public trust, staff resistance, ethical/regulatory ambiguity, and cost are socio-technical alignment problems, not merely technical deficits.

The ethics and trust items reinforce that acceptance depends on governance choices as much as on technical performance. Respondents want humans in the loop, robust privacy and data governance, transparency/explainability, and explicit accountability. They also worry about loss of human touch and algorithmic bias, indicating that managerial communication and ethical assurance are prerequisites for legitimacy. These preferences align tightly with EU Trustworthy AI requirements and suggest that hospital adoption strategies should be framed as responsible innovation programs, not technology purchases.

2.6.10 Managerial Implications

From a managerial standpoint, the findings suggest a need for a gradual, structured, and ethically guided integration of humanoid robots into healthcare systems. Managers should stage the implementation journey by prioritizing administrative and logistical applications or other non-critical workflows where the potential for early operational gains and low ethical risk is greatest. Such a phased approach allows organizations to demonstrate tangible value and build confidence before expanding robot use into more sensitive, patient-facing contexts, where trust and professional competencies must first mature.

To enhance adoption, healthcare leaders should engineer ease-of-use from the outset by investing in workflow co-design, system interoperability, and targeted staff training. Establishing "super-users" and integrating structured change-management strategies can further reduce implementation barriers and improve PEOU, which remains one of the strongest predictors of acceptance within the TAM (Davis, 1989; Venkatesh & Davis, 2000).

Equally important is the need to build trust by design by ensuring that ethical and transparency mechanisms are incorporated into system architecture from the outset. This includes establishing clear human oversight procedures, maintaining audit trails, ensuring model explainability, and upholding robust data-protection standards in compliance with the EU's Ethics Guidelines for Trustworthy AI (European Commission, 2019). Communicating these safeguards to both healthcare professionals and patients reinforces confidence and mitigates the sense of vulnerability frequently associated with AI-driven care.

At the organizational level, managers must address social legitimacy by actively involving clinicians, patients, and ethics or quality assurance teams in pilot design and evaluation. Sharing transparent outcome dashboards and key performance metrics can make both the benefits and risks of robot deployment observable to stakeholders, thereby supporting diffusion and acceptance as predicted by the DoI framework (Rogers, 2003).

Financially, managers should adopt a selective investment strategy based on a portfolio approach, allocating resources toward areas demonstrating a clear ROI, minimal ethical risk, and strong alignment with existing workflows, while discontinuing or rescoping pilots that fail to meet these criteria. Such pragmatism supports the responsible use of organizational budgets while fostering sustainable innovation.

Finally, long-term success depends on educating for governance. Managerial and leadership programs should integrate dedicated modules on AI ethics, risk management, and operational oversight, building internal capacities to manage algorithmic accountability, vendor compliance, and responsible AI deployment. This knowledge will empower future healthcare leaders to balance innovation with responsibility, aligning human-centric management principles (Maak & Pless, 2006; Voegtlin et al., 2012) with the technological realities of digital healthcare transformation.

In sum, managerial acceptance of humanoid robots in healthcare depends not only on technological performance but also on the institution's ability to govern innovation ethically, inclusively, and strategically.

2.6.11 Policy and Education Implications

Universities and professional bodies should extend AI and robotics curricula beyond technical awareness to include responsible management, health data law, safety and human-factors engineering, and evaluation methods for robot-enabled care. Educational programs should also provide opportunities for experiential learning through simulations, case studies, interdisciplinary projects, and interactions with AI-enabled technologies. Such activities can strengthen understanding of the practical, ethical, and organizational challenges associated with humanoid robots in healthcare while supporting the development of responsible leadership competencies.

Health systems and regulators can accelerate safe adoption by issuing pragmatic guidance on oversight roles, documentation standards, and post-deployment monitoring, thereby reducing uncertainty identified by respondents. Policymakers should also promote human-centric AI governance by establishing clear frameworks for accountability, transparency, patient safety, and human oversight. Consistent regulatory guidance can help healthcare organizations balance innovation with ethical responsibility, fostering greater trust among healthcare professionals, patients, and the wider public.

2.6.12 Limitations and Future Research

The sample represents individuals preparing for managerial roles, which supports external validity for emerging leadership cohorts but not for all incumbent decision-makers. Self-report measures may overstate intention relative to behavior. Future research should (1) replicate with multistakeholder samples (executives, clinicians, patients), (2) pair surveys with field experiments/pilots to measure realized outcomes (safety, quality, cost), (3) test interventions that raise PEOU (training, workflow redesign) and trust (explainability, oversight protocols), and (4) develop maturity models that sequence capabilities from supportive to patient-facing roles.

REFERENCES

Alalwan, A. A., Dwivedi, Y. K., & Rana, N. P. (2017). Factors influencing adoption of mobile banking by Jordanian bank customers: Extending UTAUT2 with trust. *International Journal of Information Management, 37*(3), 99–110.

Baxter, G., & Sommerville, I. (2011). Socio-technical systems: From design methods to systems engineering. *Interacting with Computers, 23*(1), 4–17. https://doi.org/10.1016/j.intcom.2010.07.003

Berwick, D. M. (2003). Disseminating innovations in health care. *JAMA, 289*(15), 1969–1975. https://doi.org/10.1001/jama.289.15.1969

Coeckelbergh, M. (2020). *AI Ethics*. MIT Press.

Coeckelbergh, M. (2025). Three challenges for a global AI ethics: Towards a more relational normative vision. *AI and Ethics*. Advance online publication. https://doi.org/10.1007/s43681-025-00791-9

Cresswell, K., & Sheikh, A. (2013). Organizational issues in the implementation and adoption of health information technology innovations: An interpretative review. *International Journal of Medical Informatics, 82*(5), e73–e86. https://doi.org/10.1016/j.ijmedinf.2012.10.007

Davis, F. D. (1989). Perceived usefulness, perceived ease of use, and user acceptance of information technology. *MIS Quarterly, 13*(3), 319–340.

Davis, F. D., Bagozzi, R. P., & Warshaw, P. R. (1989). User acceptance of computer technology: A comparison of two theoretical models. *Management Science, 35*(8), 982–1003.

European Commission (2019). *Ethics Guidelines for Trustworthy AI*. High-Level Expert Group on AI.

European Commission (2021). *Proposal for a Regulation laying down harmonised rules on Artificial Intelligence (AI Act).*

Floridi, L., Cowls, J., Beltrametti, M., Chatila, R., Chazerand, P., Dignum, V., Luetge, C., Madelin, R., Pagallo, U., Rossi, F., Schafer, B., Valcke, P., & Vayena, E. (2018). AI4People: An ethical framework for a good AI society. Opportunities, Risks, Principles, and Recommendations. *Minds and Machines*, *28*(4), 689–707.

Fox, W. M. (1995). Sociotechnical system principles and guidelines: Past and present. *The Journal of Applied Behavioral Science, 31*(1), 91–105. https://doi.org/10.1177/0021886395311009

Friedman, B., & Hendry, D. (2019). *Value sensitive design: Shaping technology with moral imagination.* MIT Press.

Greenhalgh, T., Robert, G., Macfarlane, F., Bate, P., & Kyriakidou, O. (2004). Diffusion of innovations in service organizations: Systematic review and recommendations. *The Milbank Quarterly*, *82*(4), 581–629. https://doi.org/10.1111/j.0887-378X.2004.00325.x

Holden, R. J., & Karsh, B. T. (2010). The Technology Acceptance Model: Its past and its future in health care. *Journal of Biomedical Informatics, 43*(1), 159–172. DOI: 10.1016/j.jbi.2009.07.002

Legris, P., Ingham, J., & Collerette, P. (2003). Why do people use information technology? A critical review of the Technology Acceptance Model. *Information & Management, 40*(3), 191–204.

Maak, T., & Pless, N. M. (2006). Responsible leadership in a stakeholder society – a relational perspective. *Journal of Business Ethics, 66*(1), 99–115.

Maillet, É., Mathieu, L., & Sicotte, C. (2015). Modeling factors explaining the acceptance, actual use and satisfaction of nurses using an electronic patient record in acute care settings: An extension of the UTAUT. *International Journal of Medical Informatics, 84*(1), 36–47. https://doi.org/10.1016/j.ijmedinf.2014.09.004

Pasmore, W. A. (1988) *Designing effective organizations: The sociotechnical systems perspective*. Wiley.

Rahimi, B., Nadri, H., Lotfnezhad Afshar, H., & Timpka, T. (2018). A systematic review of the Technology Acceptance Model in health informatics. *Applied Clinical Informatics, 9*(3), 604–634. DOI: 10.1055/s-0038-1668091

Rogers, E. (2003). *Diffusion of innovations* (5th ed.). Free Press.

Rogers, E. M. (1962). *Diffusion of innovations* (3rd ed.). Free Press.

Scarbrough, H., & Kyratsis, Y. (2022). From spreading to embedding innovation in health care: Implications for theory and practice. *Health Care Management Review, 47*(3), 236–244. https://doi.org/10.1097/HMR.0000000000000323

Siau, K., & Wang, W. (2018). Building trust in artificial intelligence, machine learning, and robotics. *Cutter Business Technology Journal, 31*(2), 47–53. https://ink.library.smu.edu.sg/sis_research/9371

Skubis, I. (2024). The EU guidelines on roboethics and ethics of sex robots. In: Lütge, C., Kriebitz, A., Max, R., & Corrigan, C. (Eds.), *The Elgar companion to applied AI ethics* (pp. 397–409). Edward Elgar Publishing.

Skubis, I. (2025a). AI and leadership in the age of automation: A critical analysis of Generation Z's perspectives on humanoid robot leaders. *International Journal of Humanoid Robotics, 22(5),* 2550006. https://doi.org/10.1142/S0219843625500069

Skubis, I. (2025b). Exploring the potential and perceptions of social robots in tourism and hospitality: Insights from industry executives and technology evaluation. *International Journal of Social Robotics*, *17*, 59–72. https://doi.org/10.1007/s12369-024-01197-z

Skubis, I. (2025c). AI governance: Ethics of trustworthy AI in healthcare. In: *Proceedings of the International Joint Conference on Neural Networks (IJCNN 2025).*

Skubis, I., Mesjasz-Lech, A., & Nowakowska-Grunt, J. (2024). Humanoid robots in tourism and hospitality – Exploring managerial, ethical, and societal challenges. *Applied Sciences*, *14*(24), 11823. https://doi.org/10.3390/app142411823

Skubis, I., & Wodarski, K. (2023). Humanoid robots in managerial positions – decision-making process and human oversight. *Scientific Papers of Silesian University of Technology*, *189*, 573–596. DOI: http://dx.doi.org/10.29119/1641-3466.2023.189.36

Trist, E., & Murray, H. (1993). *The social engagement of social science: A Tavistock anthology, Vol. II: The Socio-technical perspective.* University of Pennsylvania Press.

Trist, E. L., & Bamforth, K. W. (1951). Some social and psychological consequences of the longwall method of coal-getting: An examination of the psychological situation and defences of a work group in relation to the social structure and technological content of the work system. *Human Relations*, *4*(1), 3–38. https://doi.org/10.1177/001872675100400101

Tubaishat, A. (2017). Perceived usefulness and perceived ease of use of electronic health records among nurses: Application of Technology Acceptance Model. *Informatics for Health & Social Care*, *43*(4), 379–389. https://doi.org/10.1080/17538157.2017.1363761

Venkatesh, V., & Bala, H. (2008). Technology Acceptance Model 3 and a research agenda on interventions. *Decision Sciences, 39*(2), 273–315. https://doi.org/10.1111/j.1540-5915.2008.00192.x

Venkatesh, V., & Davis, F. D. (2000). A theoretical extension of the Technology Acceptance Model: Four longitudinal field studies. *Management Science, 46*(2), 186–204.

Voegtlin, C., Patzer, M., & Scherer, A. G. (2012). Responsible leadership in global business: A new approach to leadership and its multi-level outcomes. *Journal of Business Ethics, 105*(1), 1–16. https://doi.org/10.1007/s10551-011-0952-4

Wirtz, B. W., Weyerer, J. C., & Geyer, C. (2018). Artificial intelligence and the public sector – Applications and challenges. *International Journal of Public Administration, 42*(7), 596–615. https://doi.org/10.1080/01900692.2018.1498103

Yarbrough, A. K., & Smith, T. B. (2007). Technology acceptance among physicians: A new take on TAM. *Medical Care Research and Review, 64*(6), 650–672. DOI: 10.1177/1077558707305942

The Human-Centric Robot Acceptance Index (HCRAI)

3

The adoption of humanoid and social robots in healthcare cannot be adequately explained through purely technical or efficiency-based models. While traditional innovation and technology acceptance frameworks emphasize usefulness, usability, and performance, healthcare robotics introduces additional layers of ethical sensitivity, professional responsibility, patient vulnerability, and governance requirements. As a result, acceptance in this domain is not unidimensional but structurally conditional.

The empirical findings presented earlier in this book demonstrate that future healthcare managers do not evaluate humanoid robots solely in terms of functional benefit. Instead, their acceptance judgments are shaped by trust, ethical concern, oversight expectations, perceived patient safety, and willingness to allocate organizational resources. These factors jointly determine whether robotic systems are viewed as legitimate and adoptable components of healthcare delivery.

To capture this multidimensional structure, this chapter introduces the Human-Centric Robot Acceptance Index (HCRAI) – A Multidimensional Measure of Managerial and Ethical Readiness for Humanoid Robots in Healthcare – a composite conceptual index designed to measure readiness for humanoid robot adoption in healthcare management. The HCRAI integrates technological, ethical, governance, managerial, and patient-centered dimensions into a unified evaluative model. Its purpose is both analytical and practical: to support research comparability and to provide managers with a structured readiness assessment tool.

 DOI: 10.1201/9781042027200-4

3.1 LIMITATIONS OF SINGLE-DIMENSION ACCEPTANCE MEASURES

Most established acceptance models originate from information systems and innovation research. The Technology Acceptance Model (TAM) and its extensions focus primarily on perceived usefulness and perceived ease of use as predictors of behavioral intention. While TAM has proven highly robust across domains, healthcare robotics presents additional acceptance drivers that extend beyond performance expectations.

First, healthcare technologies operate in high-risk, high-responsibility environments where errors carry serious consequences. Second, patient interaction introduces emotional and relational dimensions absent from most enterprise IT systems. Third, regulatory and ethical governance plays a far more central role in healthcare than in many other sectors. Fourth, managerial adoption decisions involve organizational legitimacy, not only user preference.

Empirical results from the present study confirm these limitations. Respondents may rate robots as moderately useful yet remain hesitant to support implementation due to ethical concerns or lack of oversight assurance. Conversely, acceptance increases when supervision and governance mechanisms are visible, even if usability expectations remain moderate. This divergence indicates that acceptance is structurally multidimensional and cannot be reduced to technical perception alone.

The HCRAI is proposed as a response to this multidimensionality.

3.2 CONCEPTUAL FOUNDATION OF THE HCRAI

The HCRAI is grounded in a human-centric management perspective that treats technology adoption as a socio-technical and ethical decision process rather than a purely instrumental one. It integrates four theoretical streams discussed earlier in this book:

1. Technology acceptance theory (performance and usability expectations)
2. Trust and ethical AI governance frameworks
3. Socio-Technical Systems Theory
4. Responsible and human-centric management

Building on these theoretical foundations and the empirical findings presented in Chapter 2, we propose five key acceptance dimensions that together constitute the HCRAI. The proposed dimensions reflect the technological, ethical, governance, managerial, and patient-centered factors that emerged as central determinants of readiness for humanoid robot adoption in healthcare settings.

Each dimension represents a necessary condition for the responsible, ethical, and scalable adoption of humanoid robots in healthcare. Rather than viewing acceptance as a single attitude or behavioral intention, the HCRAI conceptualizes acceptance as a multidimensional construct shaped by interrelated technological, organizational, ethical, and social considerations.

Acceptance is therefore modeled not as a single attitude but as a profile across five domains. Weakness in any domain constrains adoption readiness, even if other domains score highly.

We propose that readiness for humanoid robot adoption should be assessed across these five dimensions simultaneously, as strengths in one area cannot fully compensate for substantial deficiencies in another. For example, high perceived usefulness may not translate into implementation support when ethical trust is low, governance mechanisms are absent, or patient safety concerns remain unresolved.

Building on this conceptual foundation, we propose five interrelated acceptance dimensions that collectively operationalize managerial, organizational, and ethical readiness for humanoid robot adoption in healthcare settings:

3.2.1 Dimension A: Technical Acceptance

The first dimension captures classical technology acceptance expectations. It reflects whether humanoid robots are perceived as capable of improving healthcare services and whether staff are expected to adapt to them without excessive difficulty.

Conceptual indicators include:

- Perceived usefulness for healthcare improvement
- Perceived ease of adaptation for staff

This dimension corresponds most directly to TAM constructs. It answers the question: *Is the technology seen as functionally worthwhile and usable?*

Technical acceptance represents the foundational layer of adoption readiness because healthcare organizations are unlikely to support technologies that are perceived as ineffective, difficult to use, or disruptive to existing workflows. Perceptions of usefulness and ease of use influence expectations regarding operational efficiency, quality of care, and successful implementation. However, in healthcare settings, favorable technical evaluations alone do not guarantee adoption, as ethical, governance, managerial, and patient-centered considerations also shape decision-making.

However, in the HCRAI model, technical acceptance is necessary but not sufficient.

3.2.2 Dimension B: Ethical Trust

The second dimension measures moral and reliability confidence in humanoid robots. Healthcare adoption depends strongly on whether decision-makers perceive robotic systems as ethically acceptable and behaviorally trustworthy.

Conceptual indicators include:

- Trust in robots providing care
- Intensity of ethical concerns (privacy, bias, loss of human touch, dependency, displacement)

In index logic, ethical concern operates as an inverse factor: higher concern lowers ethical trust readiness. This dimension reflects whether the technology is perceived as morally and socially acceptable, not merely efficient.

In healthcare, trust extends beyond confidence in technical performance and includes expectations regarding fairness, transparency, privacy protection, accountability, and respect for human dignity. Ethical trust is particularly important in contexts involving vulnerable patients and sensitive health information, where concerns about bias, depersonalization of care, or inappropriate decision-making may undermine acceptance. Consequently, this dimension assesses whether humanoid robots are perceived as compatible with the ethical values and social expectations that underpin healthcare practice.

3.2.3 Dimension C: Governance Assurance

The third dimension captures the role of oversight and supervision. Findings from this study show that acceptance is frequently conditional on human oversight. Governance assurance therefore forms an independent acceptance driver.

Conceptual indicators include:

- Importance assigned to human oversight
- Willingness to accept robot involvement under human supervision

This dimension does not measure trust alone but **trust-with-structure**. It reflects whether acceptance depends on defined accountability and supervision mechanisms. While Ethical Trust (Dimension B) focuses on confidence in the robot itself and concerns regarding its ethical use, Governance Assurance examines confidence in the organizational and regulatory safeguards surrounding its deployment. In other words, respondents may trust a robot's capabilities only when clear oversight procedures, human supervision, accountability arrangements, and decision-making responsibilities are in place. This dimension therefore captures the extent to which acceptance depends on governance structures that ensure responsible and transparent use of humanoid robots in healthcare.

3.2.4 Dimension D: Managerial Adoption Commitment

The fourth dimension measures organizational intention rather than personal attitude. It reflects whether respondents support institutional integration and resource allocation.

Conceptual indicators include:

- Support for robot integration in healthcare management
- Willingness to allocate resources for implementation

This dimension translates perception into strategic intention and distinguishes passive acceptance from active managerial support. Unlike technical acceptance or ethical trust, managerial adoption commitment captures the willingness to transform positive perceptions into organizational action. In healthcare settings, adoption depends not only on whether decision-makers view humanoid robots favorably, but also on whether they are prepared to invest financial, human, and organizational resources in implementation. Consequently, this dimension reflects the transition from individual evaluation to institutional commitment and strategic decision-making.

3.2.5 Dimension E: Patient Safety Perception

The fifth dimension captures perceived patient impact. Healthcare technologies are evaluated not only by operational value but by their effect on patient safety and vulnerability.

Conceptual indicators include:

- Whether patients are expected to feel safer or more vulnerable with robot assistance

This dimension introduces a patient-centered constraint on adoption readiness. Even technically effective systems face resistance if perceived to increase patient vulnerability. In healthcare settings, perceptions of safety extend beyond physical harm and encompass psychological comfort, trust, dignity, and the quality of human interaction. Consequently, acceptance of humanoid robots depends not only on their technical performance but also on whether their presence is perceived as supporting or undermining patient well-being. This dimension therefore reflects the extent to which adoption decisions are aligned with human-centric healthcare principles that prioritize patient welfare and quality of care.

3.3 HCRAI READINESS PROFILES

Instead of producing a single scalar score, the HCRAI is best interpreted through **readiness profiles**. Profile-based interpretation aligns with socio-technical assessment logic and avoids false precision.

Five ideal-type profiles can be defined:

Profile 1: Low Readiness
Low technical acceptance, low trust, high ethical concern, weak oversight confidence, low managerial support. Adoption unlikely.

Profile 2: Technically Open, Ethically Resistant
Usefulness recognized, but ethical and trust barriers dominate. Adoption blocked by legitimacy concerns.

Profile 3: Conditional Human-Centric Acceptance
Moderate usefulness and trust, strong demand for oversight, selective managerial support. Adoption possible under supervision.

Profile 4: Governance-Aligned Readiness
Strong oversight acceptance, solid trust, managerial support present. Adoption suitable in supervised roles.

Profile 5: High Human-Centric Readiness
High scores across all five dimensions. Suitable for scaled, governance-integrated adoption.

The empirical pattern observed in this study most closely aligns with **Profiles 3–4**, indicating conditional but actionable readiness.

3.4 APPLICATION FOR HEALTHCARE MANAGERS

For healthcare leaders, the HCRAI functions as a structured diagnostic tool. Before launching robot initiatives, managers can assess organizational readiness across the five dimensions.

Practical uses include:

1. Pre-pilot readiness assessment
2. Departmental comparison
3. Stakeholder perception mapping
4. Governance gap identification
5. Training and communication targeting

For example, low technical acceptance suggests training and demonstration needs, while low governance assurance suggests oversight design gaps. Low patient safety perception indicates a need for communication and pilot transparency.

3.5 RESEARCH APPLICATIONS AND THEORETICAL IMPLICATIONS

For researchers, the HCRAI offers a replicable multidimensional acceptance model tailored to healthcare robotics. It supports:

- Cross-study comparison
- Longitudinal readiness tracking
- Multi-stakeholder acceptance mapping
- Integration with TAM extensions
- Governance–trust interaction studies

Because the index is dimension-based, it can be adapted to different healthcare systems and regulatory environments while preserving conceptual structure.

The HCRAI supports three broader theoretical claims developed in this book:

- First, robot acceptance in healthcare is structurally multidimensional and governance-dependent.
- Second, ethical and oversight factors function as primary adoption drivers rather than secondary modifiers.
- Third, managerial readiness must be modeled separately from user comfort and technical perception.

These implications extend acceptance theory toward a human-centric, governance-aware model suitable for high-stakes socio-technical systems.

3.6 CONCLUSIONS

The HCRAI provides a structured and multidimensional method for understanding and measuring readiness for humanoid robot adoption in healthcare. Rather than treating acceptance as a single attitude based only on usefulness or usability, the index captures five interacting domains: technical expectations, ethical trust, governance assurance, managerial commitment, and patient safety perception. This broader structure corresponds more closely to how real adoption decisions are made in healthcare organizations, where responsibility, legitimacy, and risk perception play roles equal to performance and efficiency.

The empirical patterns discussed in this book show that decision-makers evaluate humanoid robots through conditional reasoning. Acceptance depends not only on what the technology can do, but under what safeguards, under whose supervision, and with what consequences for patients and professionals. The index makes these conditional layers visible and measurable. It therefore helps explain why technologies that appear functionally promising may still encounter hesitation, delay, or rejection in practice.

From a theoretical perspective, the index expands acceptance research by formally including governance and ethical assurance as primary dimensions rather than secondary modifiers. In healthcare robotics, oversight expectations, accountability clarity, and perceived patient impact are not peripheral concerns; they are central acceptance drivers. The index gives these drivers equal analytical status with perceived usefulness and ease of use. This provides a more realistic model of acceptance in high-stakes socio-technical environments.

From a managerial perspective, the index functions as a diagnostic instrument. It allows leaders to identify where readiness is strong and where barriers remain. Low technical scores indicate a need for demonstration and training. Low ethical trust scores indicate unresolved moral or social concerns. Low governance assurance scores reveal missing oversight structures. Low patient safety perception signals reputational and relational risk. In this way, the index supports targeted managerial action rather than generic adoption strategies.

The index also supports staged adoption planning. Because readiness is expressed as a profile across dimensions, organizations can proceed with limited, supervised, low-risk deployments even when full readiness is not yet present. This aligns with the empirical finding of conditional acceptance and supervised adoption preferences. It also supports responsible innovation principles by linking adoption speed to governance and trust conditions.

For research, the HCRAI offers a reproducible conceptual framework that can be applied across studies and settings. It enables comparison between stakeholder groups, institutions, and national contexts. It also opens a path for quantitative operationalization and future validation studies. Researchers can refine weighting schemes, test predictive power, and examine how readiness profiles change over time as exposure and experience grow.

Most importantly, the index clarifies that humanoid robot adoption in healthcare is not a purely technical decision. It is a human, organizational, and ethical decision supported by technology. By providing a structured model that reflects this reality, the HCRAI stands as one of the central analytical contributions of this book and a foundation for future research and managerial practice in responsible healthcare robotics.

4 The Risk Gradient Model of Humanoid Robot Task Acceptance in Healthcare

Acceptance of humanoid and social robots in healthcare is often discussed in general terms, as if professionals and managers either support or oppose the technology as a whole. Such a generalized perspective, however, does not reflect how adoption decisions are actually formed. Empirical evidence from this study shows that acceptance is not uniform across robot functions. Instead, it varies in a systematic and interpretable way depending on the type of task a robot is expected to perform.

Respondents distinguish clearly between administrative, technical, relational, and diagnostic uses of humanoid robots. Their willingness to accept robot involvement changes across these domains according to perceived risk, responsibility, emotional sensitivity, and possible consequences of error. This variation follows a recognizable pattern rather than random fluctuation. Understanding this pattern is essential for both theory and practice, because implementation strategies based on "robots in healthcare" as a single category overlook the internal structure of acceptance.

Based on the empirical findings of this study, we propose the Risk Gradient Model of Humanoid Robot Task Acceptance, which explains how acceptance changes across healthcare task categories and why this variation is predictable. The model shows that acceptance decreases as perceived task

DOI: 10.1201/9781042027200-5

risk, decision authority, and relational depth increase. It provides a conceptual explanation and a managerial planning tool for staged, responsible robot adoption in healthcare settings.

4.1 EMPIRICAL PATTERN OF TASK-DEPENDENT ACCEPTANCE AND THE RISK GRADIENT PRINCIPLE

The survey underlying this book did not focus solely on general attitudes toward humanoid robots in healthcare. In addition to measuring overall trust, ethical concerns, and managerial support, it examined comfort levels across specific categories of healthcare tasks. Respondents were asked how comfortable they would feel if a humanoid robot provided general medical information, conducted routine measurements, handled administrative support activities, offered social companionship for elderly patients, or delivered diagnostic or advisory recommendations. This task-level approach makes it possible to observe not only whether robots are accepted but also under which functional conditions acceptance increases or decreases.

The distribution of responses across these task categories reveals a stable and interpretable ordering. Comfort is highest when robots are assigned administrative and organizational responsibilities, such as scheduling or information management. Acceptance remains relatively strong for routine measurement and standardized technical support tasks that follow clear protocols. It becomes moderate when robots are positioned as providers of general medical information, where correctness and clarity of communication become more salient. Acceptance becomes divided when robots are described in relational and companionship roles that involve emotional or social interaction. It is lowest when robots are assigned diagnostic or decision-oriented functions that influence clinical judgment and treatment direction. This ordering appears consistently across responses and corresponds with related findings in the dataset concerning trust levels, the importance assigned to human oversight, and perceptions of patient vulnerability.

Such a pattern indicates that respondents apply differentiated evaluation criteria depending on task type. Their judgments are not driven by a symbolic reaction to "robots in healthcare" as a general concept but by a structured assessment of the specific role robots play within care processes. Delegation is viewed as more acceptable where consequences are limited and supervision is straightforward and less acceptable where outcomes are critical and responsibility is difficult to transfer. Acceptance therefore follows a logic of conditional delegation rather than categorical approval or rejection. This distinction is essential for correct interpretation of acceptance data and for realistic implementation planning.

Based on these empirical observations, we propose the central principle of the Risk Gradient Model: acceptance of humanoid robot involvement decreases as task-related risk and responsibility increase. More precisely, acceptance tends to decline when several factors intensify at the same time: the severity of potential harm if the robot fails, the degree of autonomous decision authority involved, the emotional and relational intimacy of the interaction, and the difficulty of reversing negative outcomes. These factors jointly shape how safe, appropriate, and legitimate robot involvement is perceived to be.

Administrative mistakes can usually be corrected quickly and rarely threaten patient well-being. Errors in scheduling or navigation may cause inconvenience but seldom produce lasting harm. Diagnostic errors, by contrast, can lead to delayed treatment, inappropriate intervention, or missed warning signs, with consequences that may be serious and not easily reversible. Relational failures in emotionally sensitive contexts can damage dignity, trust, and psychological comfort. It is therefore coherent, not contradictory, that the same individual expresses strong support for robots in administrative coordination while expressing hesitation toward robot-led diagnosis or advisory decisions. The gradient observed in acceptance reflects proportional risk judgment and responsibility awareness rather than inconsistency of attitude.

This interpretation places acceptance within a risk-management logic that is already familiar in healthcare governance and clinical decision-making. Healthcare technologies are routinely evaluated not only according to their capabilities but also according to consequence structure, failure impact, and oversight requirements. The Risk Gradient Model applies this same evaluative logic to humanoid robot roles. By doing so, it clarifies that task-dependent acceptance is a rational and structured response pattern. It also provides a conceptual bridge between empirical acceptance data and managerial decision frameworks for staged, responsible adoption.

4.2 THE FIVE TASK LEVELS OF THE ACCEPTANCE GRADIENT

The proposed Risk Gradient Model extends traditional technology acceptance approaches by suggesting that acceptance is not only determined by perceptions of usefulness, ease of use, trust, or governance but also by the nature of the task delegated to the technology. In healthcare, acceptance varies systematically according to perceived risk, responsibility, and relational sensitivity. Consequently, adoption should be understood not only as a question of whether a technology is accepted but also of which functions are considered appropriate for delegation to humanoid robots.

To operationalize the Risk Gradient Model, we propose five task levels that reflect increasing degrees of clinical consequence, decision authority, and ethical sensitivity. These levels form a practical classification scheme for planning humanoid robot adoption in healthcare organizations. They show that acceptance is closely tied to how directly a robot's actions affect patient outcomes, professional responsibility, and the relational core of care. Each level is associated with a distinct acceptance profile, governance requirement, and implementation strategy.

4.2.1 Level 1: Administrative and Logistical Tasks

This level includes scheduling, registration support, and navigation assistance within healthcare facilities, queue management, and routine document handling. These functions are organizational rather than clinical. They support the care process but do not directly influence diagnosis, treatment, or patient safety decisions. Because the clinical consequence is low, perceived risk remains minimal. Errors at this level are usually visible, quickly detectable, and easily reversible. Responsibility also remains clearly anchored in human staff and institutional procedures.

Acceptance at this level is typically highest because delegation does not threaten core professional roles or ethical expectations. Respondents tend to view these uses as efficiency-enhancing rather than care-replacing. From a managerial perspective, this level offers the safest and most strategically sound entry point for humanoid robot deployment. It allows organizations to introduce robotic systems in visible but low-risk roles, build staff familiarity, test technical reliability, and develop maintenance and oversight routines. Early positive experiences at this level can support broader organizational openness toward later, more advanced applications.

4.2.2 Level 2: Routine Measurement and Standardized Technical Support

This level covers tasks such as measuring vital signs, conducting basic protocol-driven check-ups, collecting standard patient parameters, and assisting with repetitive technical procedures. These activities have clinical relevance but follow clearly defined rules and thresholds. They are characterized by standardization, repeatability, and limited interpretive freedom. Risk is higher than in administrative functions but still bounded by protocol and verification possibilities.

Acceptance remains relatively high at this level, though it becomes more conditional. Respondents are generally comfortable with robot involvement when human professionals remain available to supervise results, verify anomalies, and intervene when needed. Trust is linked to device accuracy, calibration reliability, and transparency of measurement processes. From an implementation standpoint, this level is well suited for supervised pilot projects in controlled environments. Continuous monitoring, parallel human verification, and clear fallback procedures are essential. Managerially, this level supports data collection on performance and user interaction while still maintaining strong safety margins.

4.2.3 Level 3: Information and Instruction Provision

At this level, humanoid robots provide general medical information, procedural explanations, medication reminders, discharge instructions, and other forms of standardized guidance. These tasks rely heavily on communication quality, contextual appropriateness, and linguistic clarity. They do not directly intervene in the patient's body but influence understanding, expectations, and behavior. The main risk here lies in misinformation, misunderstanding, or inappropriate generalization.

Acceptance at this level is moderate and more sensitive to trust and credibility factors. Respondents often show openness to receiving routine information from robots but express caution about accuracy and contextual nuance. The tolerance for error is lower than in administrative domains because misleading information can indirectly affect patient decisions. Successful use at this level requires strict content validation, bounded knowledge domains, and explicit disclosure of the robot's informational limits. Human clarification must be easily accessible. Managerial oversight should focus on content governance, update control, and escalation pathways when questions exceed predefined knowledge scope.

4.2.4 Level 4: Relational and Companionship Roles

This level includes social interaction with elderly or isolated patients, motivational dialogue, adherence support, and companionship-oriented engagement. Direct clinical risk may be limited, but emotional, psychological, and ethical sensitivity is high. These tasks touch the relational dimension of healthcare, where empathy, dignity, and authenticity are central values. The robot is no longer only a tool but becomes a perceived social actor within the care environment.

Acceptance at this level becomes divided and often polarized. Some decision-makers and future managers recognize potential benefits, particularly in contexts of staff shortage, loneliness among patients, and the need for continuous engagement. Others express concern that relational delegation may weaken human connection, reduce perceived dignity, or create artificial substitutes for genuine care relationships. Ethical interpretation strongly influences acceptance. Implementation at this level requires careful ethical framing, explicit patient consent, transparency about the robot's non-human status, and positioning as a supplement to, not a replacement for, human interaction. Evaluation should include psychosocial outcomes and patient experience indicators, not only operational metrics.

4.2.5 Level 5: Diagnostic and Decision-Oriented Roles

This highest level includes triage suggestions, diagnostic assessments, risk stratification outputs, and treatment recommendations generated or communicated by humanoid robots. These tasks combine high consequence with interpretive authority. They influence clinical decisions and may alter treatment pathways. The potential harm associated with error is significant, and accountability questions become central.

Acceptance is lowest at this level across respondent groups. Strong hesitation appears unless strict and visible human oversight is guaranteed. Concerns focus on responsibility attribution, bias in algorithmic reasoning, transparency of decision logic, and patient safety exposure. Respondents tend to view diagnostic judgment as closely tied to professional expertise and moral accountability, which they are reluctant to delegate to autonomous systems. From a managerial perspective, this level demands the most robust governance architecture: continuous human-in-the-loop supervision, documented override authority, audit trails, and regulatory compliance checks. It is not suitable as an initial adoption stage and should only be considered when organizational readiness, oversight maturity, and legitimacy conditions are firmly established.

4.3 MANAGERIAL AND ETHICAL IMPLICATIONS OF THE GRADIENT MODEL AND ITS LINK TO READINESS ASSESSMENT

One of the most important practical consequences of the Risk Gradient Model concerns the sequencing of humanoid robot adoption in healthcare organizations. The model indicates that acceptance is structured by task-related risk and responsibility, which means that implementation strategies should follow the same structure. Adoption should proceed step by step across task levels, beginning with low-risk administrative and technical support roles and only later extending toward functions that carry higher clinical consequence and greater ethical sensitivity. In this perspective, implementation order should be guided primarily by acceptance structure and consequence exposure rather than by vendor capability, technological sophistication, or innovation pressure.

A sequenced approach offers several managerial advantages. It allows organizations to accumulate operational experience with humanoid robots under relatively safe conditions, where errors are reversible and oversight is straightforward. Early deployments in administrative and routine technical domains create opportunities to adjust workflows, clarify human–robot role boundaries, develop maintenance procedures, and establish supervision protocols. Staff training can be conducted progressively, and resistance can be addressed through direct experience rather than abstract persuasion.

Trust develops through observed reliability and transparent evaluation rather than expectation alone. In contrast, attempting immediate deployment in high-stakes diagnostic or decision-oriented roles increases the probability of professional resistance, staff rejection, patient distrust, and reputational risk. When adoption moves faster than social and ethical readiness, even technically successful systems may fail organizationally. A gradient-based sequencing logic therefore supports stability, legitimacy, and sustainable scaling.

The gradient pattern also carries important ethical meaning. Lower acceptance of high-risk and high-relational robot roles reflects professional and moral judgment about responsibility, empathy, and accountability in healthcare. Tasks that involve diagnosis, interpretive judgment, and emotionally sensitive interaction are widely regarded as requiring human presence not only for technical competence but also for moral and relational reasons. Hesitation toward robot involvement in these domains expresses concern for dignity, contextual understanding, and the quality of care relationships. It should not be interpreted as simple resistance to innovation or lack of technological openness. Rather, it signals that decision-makers apply differentiated moral thresholds depending on the nature of the task and the vulnerability of the patient situation.

Recognizing this ethical layer is essential for governance design and communication strategy. It clarifies that conditional acceptance, support for robots in some roles but not others, is compatible with a generally positive orientation toward healthcare innovation. The central question is not whether humanoid robots should be present in healthcare but in which functions, under which safeguards, and with which forms of accountability. Communication that ignores this distinction risks mischaracterizing cautious acceptance as opposition. Governance frameworks that acknowledge it can design role boundaries and oversight mechanisms that respect professional and ethical expectations while still enabling technological progress.

The Risk Gradient Model is most effective when used together with the Human-Centric Robot Acceptance Index introduced in the previous chapter. The index provides a multidimensional assessment of readiness across technical expectations, ethical trust, governance assurance, managerial commitment, and patient safety perception. It indicates how prepared an organization or stakeholder group is for humanoid robot adoption. While the HCRAI focuses on measuring readiness for humanoid robot adoption across multiple acceptance dimensions, the Risk Gradient Model focuses on the allocation of robot functions according to perceived risk, responsibility, and ethical sensitivity. The gradient model, by contrast, identifies which categories of tasks correspond to that readiness level. One model evaluates acceptance capacity across dimensions; the other maps that capacity onto appropriate functional roles. Used together, they provide both diagnostic and strategic guidance. Decision-makers can first assess readiness profiles and then select adoption entry points and expansion paths that match those profiles. This combined use strengthens human-centered planning and reduces the likelihood of a mismatch between technological ambition and organizational legitimacy.

Conclusions

This book set out to connect two domains that are often treated separately: human-centric AI as a regulatory and ethical project and human-centric AI as an organizational and managerial practice. Through the Human-Centric AI Governance Ecosystem Framework, the book demonstrated that human-centric governance must be understood across three layers: macro regulation, meso organizational implementation, and micro human experience, and that failure at any layer can undermine adoption, legitimacy, and societal trust.

The first chapter showed that the AI Act explicitly positions human-centric AI as a strategic and normative objective linked to protection of fundamental rights, health, safety, and broader public interests. The Act's recurring references to human well-being, inclusivity, user-friendliness, social and environmental well-being, gender balance, and human dignity highlight an effort to anchor innovation in values rather than purely in market efficiency or technical capability. In this sense, the AI Act provides a robust normative orientation: AI should be developed and used as a tool for people, subject to oversight, accountability, and safeguards against manipulative or exploitative practices.

The content analysis conducted in Chapter 1 demonstrated that human-centricity is not a peripheral concept within the AI Act but a recurring normative principle embedded throughout the Regulation. The analysis identified multiple references to human-centric AI, human well-being, social and environmental well-being, user-friendliness, inclusivity, gender balance, and human dignity. In particular, the notions of inclusivity and human dignity appeared repeatedly across provisions related to AI governance, high-risk systems, stakeholder participation, and fundamental rights protection. The findings suggest that the AI Act conceptualizes AI not merely as a technological innovation but as a socio-technical system that must remain aligned with human values, democratic principles, and societal well-being.

Furthermore, the analysis revealed that references to human-centric AI are consistently associated with complementary concepts such as trustworthy AI, ethical AI, human oversight, accountability, transparency, and the protection of fundamental rights. This finding indicates that the European Union does not treat human-centricity as an isolated principle but rather as an overarching governance philosophy connecting innovation, safety, ethics, and societal trust. The AI Act therefore provides not only a legal framework for AI regulation but also a normative vision of how AI should be designed, deployed, and governed in society.

The content analysis further revealed that references to inclusivity and human dignity appeared multiple times throughout the Act, while concepts such as gender balance, social and environmental well-being, and user-friendliness were also explicitly incorporated into the regulatory framework. These findings provide empirical support for the argument that the AI Act places human-centric values at the core of AI governance.

The second chapter demonstrated, however, that the presence of human-centric regulation does not automatically translate into organizational readiness. Survey findings portray conditional optimism toward humanoid robots in healthcare: perceived usefulness is moderate, perceived ease of use is lower, and support depends strongly on human oversight and ethical assurance. Respondents favor low-risk roles and selective resource allocation, while identifying public trust, ethical and regulatory uncertainty, staff resistance, and cost as major barriers. These patterns reveal that the obstacles are often socio-organizational rather than purely technical. In other words, adoption is constrained less by "what robots can do" than by "whether organizations can govern them responsibly" while preserving dignity, empathy, and trust.

The third chapter extended this discussion by introducing the Human-Centric Robot Acceptance Index (HCRAI), a multidimensional framework designed to assess readiness for humanoid robot adoption in healthcare. The HCRAI demonstrates that acceptance cannot be adequately explained through technological considerations alone. Instead, readiness emerges from the interaction of technical acceptance, ethical trust, governance assurance, managerial commitment, and patient safety perceptions. By integrating these dimensions, the framework offers both a conceptual and practical tool for evaluating organizational preparedness for human-centric AI implementation. The HCRAI therefore contributes to existing technology acceptance research by incorporating ethical and governance dimensions that are particularly important in high-stakes healthcare environments.

The fourth chapter further refined understanding of adoption dynamics through the development of the Risk Gradient Model of Humanoid Robot Task Acceptance in Healthcare. The model demonstrates that acceptance is task-dependent and varies systematically according to perceived risk, responsibility, decision authority, and relational sensitivity. Stakeholders generally express greater acceptance of humanoid robots performing administrative, logistical, and routine support functions, while demonstrating increased caution toward diagnostic, advisory, and highly relational roles. This finding suggests that successful implementation is likely to occur through gradual and staged adoption strategies rather than through broad replacement-oriented approaches.

The empirical component of the book, based on a survey of 527 management students representing future organizational decision-makers, provided evidence that attitudes toward humanoid robots in healthcare are shaped by a combination of technological, ethical, organizational, and governance-related factors. The findings revealed that acceptance is conditional upon the existence of meaningful human oversight, ethical safeguards, and confidence in organizational readiness. Public trust, regulatory and ethical uncertainty, implementation costs, and potential staff resistance emerged as key concerns influencing adoption decisions, suggesting that the future of humanoid robots in healthcare will be shaped not only by technological progress but also by organizational preparedness and governance maturity.

The study also demonstrated that acceptance varies considerably according to the nature of the healthcare task being performed. Respondents expressed greater support for humanoid robots undertaking administrative, informational, logistical, and routine support functions than for activities involving diagnosis, treatment decisions, or emotionally sensitive interactions with patients. This pattern highlights the continued importance of human judgment, empathy, and professional accountability in healthcare and provides the empirical foundation for the development of the Risk Gradient Model of Humanoid Robot Task Acceptance.

The findings revealed that respondents were generally open to the use of humanoid robots in healthcare, although this acceptance was highly conditional. While 52% expressed support for the integration of humanoid robots in hospitals and healthcare management, support was primarily directed toward low-risk applications. Nearly half of respondents (49%) identified administrative functions as the most appropriate role for humanoid robots, whereas considerably fewer supported their involvement in medical advice, monitoring, or direct patient-care activities. These results suggest a preference for complementary rather than replacement-oriented models of human–robot collaboration.

The study further demonstrated that human oversight remains a central prerequisite for acceptance. More than half of respondents (53%) considered human oversight either extremely important or very important, while 44% indicated willingness to accept robot-assisted healthcare only under human supervision. These findings reinforce the importance of maintaining human agency, accountability, and professional responsibility in healthcare environments characterized by high levels of uncertainty and ethical sensitivity.

Ethical concerns also appeared as significant determinants of acceptance. The most frequently reported concern was the potential loss of human touch in patient care (39%), followed by bias in AI decision-making (24%) and data privacy and security concerns (18%). In contrast, technological limitations were perceived as less problematic than social and organizational challenges. Indeed, lack of public trust and acceptance (71%), ethical and regulatory uncertainty (56%), staff resistance (52%), and implementation costs (50%) were identified as the most important barriers to adoption. These findings suggest that the successful integration of humanoid robots depends less on technological capability than on governance, organizational readiness, and stakeholder trust.

Furthermore, the HCRAI demonstrated that readiness for humanoid robot adoption is multidimensional and cannot be adequately explained through technological considerations alone. Acceptance emerged from the interaction of technical acceptance, ethical trust, governance assurance, managerial commitment, and patient safety perceptions. These findings underscore the importance of adopting a broader human-centric perspective when evaluating emerging technologies in healthcare environments.

Taken together, the findings from all four chapters suggest that human-centric AI governance should be understood as a continuous process rather than a static regulatory outcome. Chapter 1 demonstrated how human-centric principles are embedded within the AI Act at the regulatory level, while Chapters 2–4 illustrated the practical challenges associated with translating these principles into organizational decision-making, stakeholder acceptance, and healthcare implementation. The findings demonstrate that successful implementation depends on alignment across regulatory principles, organizational readiness, managerial capabilities, governance mechanisms, and stakeholder trust. Human-centric governance therefore depends on alignment across all levels of the socio-technical ecosystem. The findings further suggest that the human-centric principles embedded in the AI Act can serve as a foundation for responsible healthcare robotics but only when translated into concrete governance practices, organizational capabilities, and oversight mechanisms.

Moreover, the book contributes to the literature through the development of two complementary conceptual frameworks: the HCRAI and the Risk Gradient Model of Humanoid Robot Task Acceptance. Together, these models provide practical tools for assessing organizational readiness, understanding stakeholder acceptance, and designing phased implementation strategies for humanoid robots in healthcare settings. These frameworks extend existing technology acceptance and AI governance literature by integrating human-centric, ethical, managerial, and risk-based perspectives within a single analytical approach.

The book also highlights several implications. For policymakers and regulators, legal requirements benefit from operational guidance that clarifies oversight roles, documentation standards, and post-deployment monitoring in sector-specific contexts such as hospitals. For organizations, successful adoption requires socio-technical alignment: co-design with staff, workflow integration, training, and clear governance that defines responsibility and escalation pathways. For management education, the findings indicate that future leaders need competencies not only in innovation strategy but also in responsible governance, including human oversight, trust calibration, risk management, and ethical communication.

The findings also have implications for healthcare organizations seeking to implement humanoid robots and AI systems. Rather than focusing exclusively on technical performance indicators, decision-makers should evaluate organizational readiness, stakeholder perceptions, governance mechanisms, and task-specific risk profiles. Adoption strategies that acknowledge these factors are more likely to achieve sustainable implementation and long-term legitimacy.

Looking ahead, human-centric AI governance will be tested by increasingly capable systems and by ongoing pressures in healthcare systems. The pathway forward is not simply "more technology" but better governance maturity: staged adoption in low-risk roles, evidence-driven evaluation, robust oversight, and continuous trust-building with patients and professionals. If the human-centric approach is to remain credible, it must be enacted as a practical discipline of management and institutional design, ensuring that AI and robotics serve people, protect dignity, and strengthen the legitimacy of healthcare systems rather than undermining them.

Future research should further validate and refine the HCRAI and the Risk Gradient Model across different stakeholder groups, healthcare systems, and cultural contexts. Comparative studies involving healthcare professionals, patients, policymakers, and technology developers may provide additional insights into the factors that shape trust, acceptance, and responsible adoption. Such research would contribute to the development of more robust frameworks for human-centric AI governance and support evidence-based approaches to the integration of humanoid robots in healthcare.

Ultimately, the book argues that the future of AI and robotics in healthcare should not be evaluated solely in terms of technological sophistication or efficiency gains. Rather, its success will depend on whether these technologies remain aligned with human values, respect human dignity, preserve meaningful human oversight, and strengthen trust in healthcare institutions. Human-centric AI governance is therefore not merely a regulatory objective but a managerial, organizational, and societal responsibility. The long-term success of AI and humanoid robotics in healthcare will depend not only on what these technologies are capable of doing but also on whether they are implemented in ways that preserve trust, accountability, human dignity, and meaningful human oversight.

Index

For Product Safety Concerns and Information please contact our EU representative GPSR@taylorandfrancis.com
Taylor & Francis Verlag GmbH, Kaufingerstraße 24, 80331 München, Germany

www.ingramcontent.com/pod-product-compliance
Ingram Content Group UK Ltd.
Pitfield, Milton Keynes, MK11 3LW, UK
UKHW021703300926
475953UK00017B/25
* 9 7 8 1 0 4 1 4 1 3 6 4 6 *